Natural Solutions
for Digestive Health

Relief from the most common
problems including:
- Acid Reflux • IBS • Gas • Constipation
- Diarrhea • Crohn's Disease • Ulcers
- Children's Digestive Issues • and more

Dr. Jillian Sarno Teta &
Jeannette Bessinger, CHHC
Foreword by Jonny Bowden, PhD, CNS

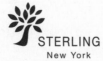
STERLING
New York

STERLING
New York

An Imprint of Sterling Publishing
387 Park Avenue South
New York, NY 10016

ISBN 978-1-4549-1031-2

Library of Congress Cataloging-in-Publication Data

Sarno Teta, Jillian.
  Natural solutions for digestive health : relief from the most common problems including : acid reflux,
IBS, gas, constipation, diarrhea, Crohn's Disease, ulcers, children's digestive issues, and more / Dr.
Jillian Sarno Teta, Jeannette L. Bessinger, CHHC ; foreword by Jonny Bowden, PhD, CNS.
    pages cm
  ISBN 978-1-4549-1031-2 (paperback)
  1. Gastrointestinal system--Diseases--Alternative treatment. 2. Naturopathy--Popular works. I.
Bessinger, Jeannette. II. Title.
  RC827.S27 2014
  616.3'3--dc23
                              2014007040

Distributed in Canada by Sterling Publishing
c/o Canadian Manda Group, 165 Dufferin Street
Toronto, Ontario, Canada M6K 3H6
Distributed in the United Kingdom by GMC Distribution Services
Castle Place, 166 High Street, Lewes, East Sussex, England BN7 1XU
Distributed in Australia by Capricorn Link (Australia) Pty. Ltd.
P.O. Box 704, Windsor, NSW 2756, Australia

For information about custom editions, special sales, and premium
and corporate purchases, please contact Sterling Special Sales at 800-805-5489
or specialsales@sterlingpublishing.com.

Manufactured in the United States of America

2 4 6 8 10 9 7 5 3

www.sterlingpublishing.com

This book is dedicated to everyone working toward greater health.

Special dedication from Jillian to you

Special dedication from Jeannette with great love
to her whole funny, fabulous family

The authors would like to thank our talented and persistent agent, Coleen O'Shea, Sterling's amazing team, and especially the lovely Jennifer Williams, our editor. We would also like to thank Dr. Sunita Iyer, ND, LM, and Kathi Kemper, MD, for their instrumental information and suggestions about pediatric digestive health.

And a very special thank-you to Dr. Jonny Bowden, unequaled nutrition expert and friend-for-life, for getting the whole process rolling and writing the fantastic foreword.

Jillian's Acknowledgments

This book would not be possible without the prior work and dedication of many brilliant individuals. Thank you to Jeffrey Bland, Liz Lipski, Alessio Fasano, Peter Green, and Tristan Biesecker for your excellence. Deep gratitude to Esther Blum for making the right connection at the right time. Jeannette, thank you for your wisdom, kindness, competence, and steady hand through this process. I have the best friends in the world that offer unwavering support, humor, and refuge—thank you Melody Stockdale, Rebecca Mexico, Gina Bangtson, Ryan Martin, Jean Paul Boisvert, Sunita Iyer, Hillary Lampers, Jaclyn Chasse, Sabrina Kimball, Julius Torelli, Julie Milunic, and Melissa Wilkey. My patients and clients are the best teachers in the world and continue to humble and amaze me. Sometimes, there are people that lovingly push you out of your comfort zone and give you wings, and I would like to thank Jill Coleman and Jade Teta for that. My family, near and far, has offered inspiration and unconditional support at every turn. My parents Ralph and Barbara, brother Marc, grandparents Joan, Frank, and Violet, in-laws Joyce and Jimmy, and many aunts, uncles, cousins, nieces, and nephews have been my backbone. Thank you Terry, Don, Joan, Kevin, Karen, Michael, Frank, Annie, Diane, Bridgit, Anna, Andrew, Kate, Kimo, Lana, Jodi, Eli, Soul, Zen, Lili, Quentin, and Alisa—you are all simply the best. And last, but certainly not least—thank you Keoni, for everything.

Jeannette's Acknowledgments

To the gorgeous paleo guru Esther Blum for introducing me to Jillian—thank you and thank you; to Jillian, you are a shining light, my friend, and I am grateful for your high expertise and easy ways, a rare combination; ongoing thanks to my beloved family for the unending laughter, and to my patient tasting crew; and finally, big love and thanks to Jay, Jesse, Julian, and the furries for your patience and support at deadline time . . . again.

Contents

Foreword

Though some people will read a great book like this just because they want to learn more about the human digestive system, many more will turn to it because of personal health issues.

The moment you pop a morsel of food into your mouth, a symphony of metabolic and enzymatic reactions begin to take place. And like any exquisitely complicated system with many moving parts, things frequently break down or go awry. That's when you notice the obvious symptoms like bloat, diarrhea, constipation, stomach upset, heartburn, or headaches.

But an impaired digestive system can produce problems that are a lot worse than those common digestive complaints (bad as they may be). When the gut isn't working right, all sorts of problems occur, some of them chronic, some of them serious, many of them problems you probably didn't realize were related to digestion in the first place.

No wonder the digestive system is becoming one of the hottest topics in natural health. The nervous system that controls digestion—known as the enteric nervous system (ENS)—also plays a critical role in how we *feel*—in both our mental and our physical well-being. This system is so vast and complex that it's been called "The Second Brain."

As a nutritionist, I've always subscribed to the mantra that good health begins with the food you put into your body. But as you'll learn from this book, that's only the beginning. It's the fate of that food that really makes the difference to your health.

That's where digestive health comes in.

The two authors of this book are uniquely qualified to take you on the journey to digestive—and ultimately, *overall-* health. Dr. Jillian Sarno Teta is a medically trained naturopathic doctor and the developer and founder of Fix Your Digestion, an online education program for restoring optimal gut health and digestive function. She's also one of the country's premiere experts in integrative gastroenterology. Jeannette Bessinger is one of the smartest, most knowledgeable health coaches on the planet. A trained chef, she is the person I've chosen to co-author five cookbooks with me, and anyone who's tried her recipes knows why. But more than that, Jeannette is a world-class educator. A natural born teacher, she's been coaching people for decades in how to make simple, easy changes that result in profound improvements in health.

To summarize: You need the information in this book. And these two powerful and knowledgeable women are uniquely qualified to deliver it.

—Jonny Bowden, PhD, CNS aka "the Rogue Nutritionist"

Introduction

What is digestion, anyway? We pop some food into our mouth, trust that our bodies know what to do with it, and forget about it until it's time to take a trip to the bathroom.

We hardly think about digestion at all unless something goes wrong in the system: heartburn, perhaps, or gas and bloating. Many are chronically constipated or plagued by loose stool. Perhaps you have been diagnosed with a digestive disorder but don't really know what it means or what you can do to help yourself. Often, we take for granted that nagging symptoms like gas, bloating, and indigestion are a "normal" part of life, when in fact they are symptoms of something deeper going on.

The purpose of this book is to help you and your digestive system feel better. Digestion can be a complicated topic, but we've broken it down for you into practical, easy-to-understand sections that will quickly get you the information you need to fix what ails you:

Section 1: "The basics of normal digestion and what can go wrong" is a tour of the gastrointestinal system and explains the "what" of the normal function of the most important gastrointestinal players and what can go wrong at each step. It's a trip down the amazing system we call the digestive tract, visiting major organs of digestion. Section II: "Modern living and the downfall of digestion" reviews the "why": a variety of ways that our modern lifestyle contributes to digestive distress and discomfort. Section III: "The Gut Restoration Program" outlines the "how" of relieving your digestive discomfort, including a twenty-eight-day meal plan and supplement schedule. This plan will empower you by helping to identify factors in your lifestyle that are contributing to your symptoms. Section IV: "Conditions" offers information, tips, and tricks that can be built into your Gut Restoration Program to fit your individual needs. Finally, Section V: "Gastrointestinal health for kids" addresses the unique digestive issues that children face and offers solutions.

This book will serve you well as a comprehensive resource. Feel free to slowly peruse the sections sequentially or dive right into the part most relevant to what ails you. It is our hope that you find the answers to your most pressing questions about digestion and, even more important, relief from your suffering.

The Basics of Normal Digestion and What Can Go Wrong

CHAPTER 1

The Process of Digestion

Digestion Fundamentals

At first glance, digestion seems simple and uncomplicated. The reality is that digestion is the multiple-step process of eating, the extraction of the nutrients from the food we have eaten, and the elimination of what is left behind. The main steps of digestion are:

- **Chewing.** The very first step of physical digestion begins in your mouth. The chicken Caesar salad you've ordered for lunch is ground by your teeth, moved around your mouth by your tongue, and mixed with saliva, making it a soft, soupy mouthful called a **bolus**. Enzymes in the saliva then begin to break down carbohydrates and sugars in your mouth (ever notice how bread or grain gets sweeter the longer it is chewed?).

- **Stoking digestive fire.** Once you start thinking about lunch and begin to eat, your brain sends signals to the stomach, pancreas, liver, and gallbladder to let them know that food is expected imminently: the stomach steps up its production of powerful hydrochloric acid (HCl) to break up protein molecules; the pancreas releases enzymes to aid in the breakdown of fats, proteins, and carbohydrates; and the gallbladder releases bile to break down fats. The term **digestive fire** describes the body's ability to produce adequate amounts of acid, enzymes, and bile to break down food into tiny constituent particles of amino acids, sugars, starches, and fatty acids. All other digestive processes hinge on this ability. Large unbroken, partially digested food molecules aren't well absorbed and can wreak body-wide havoc.

Chew Your Food

Most people don't truly chew their food. We tend to eat more like snakes than mammals and chew food just long enough to get it down our throat. On average, Americans chew each bite five to seven times. This puts more strain on the stomach, digestive enzymes, acid, and bile to break down food. If one part of the chain isn't fully doing its job, the whole drain suffers. Is it any wonder so many of us are suffering from digestive disturbances? The gut isn't built to break down large pieces of food. The act of thoroughly chewing your food is a simple, powerful, and often-overlooked strategy for improving digestion. Chewing is also a natural relaxant. This slow, rhythmic, meditative action will, over time, begin to send calming signals to your brain.

Q. How many times should you chew each bite?
A. That depends on the type of food and size of the bite. Start by taking a reasonably sized forkful rather than a giant mouthful. Proteins need to be softened or broken up thoroughly—and acid in the stomach will do the rest of the digestive work to break them down. Carbs, such as starchy vegetables and grains, on the other hand, need to be ground into a paste and thoroughly mixed with saliva for optimal digestion and maximum nutrient absorption. If you're chewing carbs, start with twenty chews per bite. To make chewing a calming practice, try for thirty-five chews. If you don't want to count your chews, just make sure that each bite you take has been reduced to a soft mash in your mouth before you swallow it. If you can roll food around in your mouth and it still feels like an almond or a piece of broccoli, you've got more chewing to do.

◉ **Transport of food.** Swallowing is the last voluntary act of digestion until you decide to go to the bathroom. The movement of the esophagus, the secretion of enzymes, acids, and bile, and all subsequent steps are under involuntary control (and it's a good thing, too! Imagine if we had to keep track of all that!). The chewed-up bolus of food in your mouth is swallowed and lands in your stomach. There, enzymes, acid, and bile await—the products of digestive fire. The stomach is not a passive receptacle, however. It is a muscular organ, and when food is present it begins to flex! The stomach churns and grinds, helping all of the digestive juices break down your lunch into itty-bitty particles. Then those food particles begin their long journey through the intestines in a process known as **peristalsis**—the rhythmic, muscular contractions that guide the food down and through the digestive tract.

○ **Absorption and assimilation.** In this step of digestion, the teensy-weensy food particles that have been thoroughly crushed and biochemically broken down interact with the lining of the small intestines. The particles are taken through the lining and into the body. It is interesting to note—and important to understand— that food does not enter your blood and is not usable for energy or nutrition until it is absorbed through the cells of the intestine. It is then transported into the blood and becomes available to the muscles, brain, and other organs. Until this happens, the food particles are resting inside the tube of the intestine, called the lumen. Once the nutrients are absorbed, they need to be assimilated into the cells. Assimilation is the uptake of amino acids, glucose, fatty acids, vitamins, minerals, and other absorbed compounds into the cells of the body.

○ **Elimination.** There is just no elegant way to talk about elimination. Elimination, of course, refers to having a bowel movement. The stool is what's left of lunch after the nutrients and water have been removed from it. The body can do no more with it, so it's dumped as waste. In addition to indigestible fibers and other food components, the stool also contains bacteria, skin cells that have sloughed off in the GI tract, and metabolic waste products. Defecation is the first voluntary digestive action after swallowing, which means you get to decide when and where to have a bowel movement (at least in a perfect world). Ignoring the signals to defecate can set up a host of troubles.

CHAPTER 2

Roles of the Digestive System

If you are not impressed yet by the humble GI tract, consider the multiple roles that it plays beyond digestion. Your gut is very busy indeed and wears quite a few unexpected hats.

The gut is the body's Grand Central Station, linking the functions of digestion and the absorption and assimilation of nutrients to every other system of the body. The endocrine system, with its complex web of hormonal signaling, interfaces with the digestive system and shapes hormonal expression, body composition, and the way we burn fuel. The majority of immune cells reside in the gastrointestinal tract, where they interact with our own cells, foreign cells, food particles, and environmental agents. The immune system is greatly influenced by what is delivered into the gut. Digestive function is tied to the nervous system. Aspects of stress, relaxation, and other input from the brain, spinal cord, and nerves greatly influence digestive function and vice versa. In fact, the gastrointestinal (GI) system has its own "brain"—the so-called second brain—in the form of some hundred million nerve cells called the **enteric nervous system** (ENS). The large intestine is one of the five major organs of detoxification and is inextricably connected to the skin, kidneys, liver, and lungs.

Defense

The gastrointestinal system is on the front lines of your body's defense against pathogenic organisms, such as harmful bacteria and yeast; toxic compounds, such as persistent organic pollutants; alcohol; and other unsavory foes. This makes good sense because most of what can harm us comes in through what we eat and swallow.

One of the body's first line of defense comes in the form of **IgA** (immunoglobulin A), a non-inflammatory immune molecule. IgA is found on all of our mucous membranes, from the mouth all the way down the GI tract and including the genitourinary tract as well. IgA attaches to harmful substances that you eat or breathe in and flags them for immune cells to examine.

Next in the line of defense is the mighty stomach and stomach acid that is so strong and the pH so low, that if it were to spill on your skin it would burn a hole. This acid does a tidy job of destroying many pathogenic organisms that you may have consumed.

The lining of the small intestine, also known as the **gut mucosa**, does more than absorb nutrients from food. It acts like a very smart filter, taking in the important nutrition and shutting out bad guys. It is an important barrier that keeps pathogenic organisms and toxic or harmful particles out.

The gastrointestinal tract is the seat of the immune system. More than two-thirds of the entire immune system lives there.

Search and Destroy

The job of the immune system is simple: find and kill **antigens**—compounds such as harmful bacteria or toxins that do not belong to the body. The immune system is absolutely ruthless and relentless in its search-and-destroy mission. It's a good thing too, because were it not for this action, you would be overwhelmed by infection in no time. The immune system uses antibodies to target, kill, or neutralize harmful substances.

This raises some questions about the immune system: Our food is not human. The bacteria that populate our guts are not human either, so what is going on? Early in infancy, as the immune system is developing, immune cells go through a process called **tolerization**, which is run primarily by the thalamus gland. During this process, immune cells are "schooled" and taught that antigens from food and native, beneficial gut flora should be tolerated and not targeted. Any immune cell that takes action against food or bacterial antigens is immediately culled. The immune system is very strict. Only immune cells that tolerate the food and bacterial antigens they are shown make the cut. These cells survive and go forth into the body and propagate their cell lines.

Tolerization can be lost through chronic stress, improper diet, injury to the digestive system, or "leaky gut" (a condition where the integrity of the lining of the small intestine is compromised). Once tolerization is lost, the stage is set for auto-immune disease to crop up via a process called **molecular mimicry**. The immune system attacks the body's tissues in autoimmune disease, which is the opposite of the system's purpose, and harmful to the body.

Molecular Mimicry and Autoimmune Disease

Molecular mimicry occurs when the immune system makes a leap from making antibodies against food particles (as in the case of food allergies/sensitivities) to making antibodies against our own tissues that have a similar "blueprint" to those food particles. Food sensitivities are created by a dysfunctional immune response that arises from a variety of factors, most of them revolving around improper nutrition and suboptimal integrity and function of the lining of the small intestine. Autoimmune responses from molecular mimicry represent the culmination of many steps that have gone awry in the digestive and immune interface.

Bacterial Allies

The microbiota, a large colony of beneficial bacteria that live in the large intestine, are a great friend of the immune cells. They help keep the immune system tolerant and calm, much in the same way as a diplomatic friend might help you navigate a rough patch. A disruption in the microbiota can lead to a disruption in the immune system. This helps explain why probiotic supplementation can help balance immune response and buffer against **autoimmunity**.

Your beneficial bacteria also aid the immune system directly by producing anti-microbial substances that kill bacteria, yeasts, and other pathogens and by simply taking up space to crowd out bad guys from setting up shop in your body. They also help neutralize compounds that are excreted by harmful bacteria and yeasts that may be lurking in your body and, in some cases, can even prevent the creation of these toxins.

The Second Brain

There is an enormous amount of nervous tissue between your esophagus and rectum, a whopping 100 million nerve cells' worth. For perspective, that is almost as many nerve cells as found in the spinal cord. This tissue is called the enteric nervous system, known as the second brain.

Typically, we humans are extremely proud of our big brain, yet it turns out that there is quite a bit of substance to the brain in our belly! Although the enteric nervous system gets input from the brain, it is capable of overriding signals and operating entirely on its own.

Actually, it's a really good thing that your digestive system has a nervous system to call its own. For practical purposes, if all of the nerve cells that are needed for digestion were stored in your head and connected to the digestive organs, the thickness of all of that tissue would be intolerable. You wouldn't even be able to bend over to tie your shoes!

There is protective wisdom in the ENS. If you did not have your second brain, a spinal cord injury would render you unable to digest food, because the cells from your brain couldn't communicate with your digestive organs. As your ability to digest is critical for survival, the body has an elegant solution—a second brain!

Having the enteric nervous system means that you do not need to put one iota of thought into your digestive process—it all happens for you. Unlike muscles that need commands in order to move, the digestive organs need no such prompting from you.

Lastly, we can take heart in that the digestive system is not competing for the brain's attention with other major functions such as breathing or temperature regulation. Quite simply, your gastrointestinal system gets to do its own thing. Although it is in communication with the brain and central nervous system, the second brain can function independently of them.

The ENS largely controls the rate at which food moves through your system on its journey from start to finish. Peristalsis, the rhythmic, muscular contraction that propels food toward its final destination, is controlled by the ENS. The ENS also has input into the amounts of digestive juice and hormones that are secreted and the rate at which they are secreted.

Digestion is not a passive, arbitrary process but a highly complex, regulated one, monitored by a system that senses its progress on a moment-to-moment basis and adjusts accordingly.

The Second Brain Plays Well with Others

The ENS receives information from the **autonomic nervous system** (ANS). The autonomic nervous system is responsible for all actions that are outside of conscious control—such as breathing, heart rate, blood pressure, etc. The ANS is then divided into two branches that may be familiar to you: the sympathetic nervous system, also known as the "fight or flight" branch, and the parasympathetic system, also known as the "rest and digest" branch. Digestion is more favorable and efficient when we are in parasympathetic mode and not stressed.

We do live in a stressful world, however. The sympathetic and parasympathetic branches of the nervous system are always in balance with each other, very much like a seesaw. However, if you are chronically stressed, and your seesaw tips in such a way as to make the sympathetic nervous system dominant, GI symptoms can crop up that were not present before. This is why stress management is so crucial.

The enteric nervous system receives input from your gut microbiota, your immune system, and central nervous system/consciousness (anyone ever tell you that you have a nervous stomach? It's a real thing . . .) along with food, drugs, and stress. All of these things can ensure smooth sailing or create problems in the GI system.

Detoxification and Digestion

Detoxification is one of those tricky words, because when some people hear it they think about special teas and diets, fasting, colon cleanses, or something special that you have to do that creates detoxification. Marketers hijacked the term in order to sell products to us, as a means to an end. Detoxification sounds very sexy and interesting when it appears in the same sentence with digestion.

Yet here is the truth: Detoxification is happening in our bodies twenty-four hours a day, seven days a week, three hundred and sixty-five days a year. Detoxification is part of the normal metabolic process. Simply put, detoxification is the process by which harmful compounds from our internal or external environment, spent hormones, and other by-products of metabolism are processed, rendered harmless (or at least less harmful), and excreted out of the body.

Can steps be taken to facilitate and optimize this process? Absolutely. By cleaning up the digestive system and restoring gut function, you will greatly aid the processes of detoxification—all without gimmicks.

The five major organs of detoxification are the liver, the large intestine, the kidneys, the skin, and the lungs. We sure do give these organs plenty to do! There are 6,000—yup, six THOUSAND—new chemicals registered *per week* in the Chemical Society's Chemical Archives, and it is estimated that the average American eats 14 pounds of food additives per year. This load is in addition to what we breathe in daily and what we slather onto our skin in the form of pthalates, parabens, triclosan, surfactants, and a variety of other synthetic and potentially harmful compounds.

What's Lurking in Your Bathroom and Laundry Room?

Pthalates and **parabens** are compounds added to many personal-care and hygiene products to increase their shelf life and improve their feel. These chemicals are also known to disrupt hormonal balance.

Triclosan is an antimicrobial agent often added to soaps and hand sanitizers. Frequent exposure of triclosan has been correlated with increased levels of allergy in children and is responsible for the development of antibiotic-resistant superbugs. Triclosan, like pthalates and parabens, can throw hormonal function off and is being studied as a potential cancer-causing agent. All products that contain triclosan are required to be labeled as such.

Surfactants are used in soaps and laundry detergent to help break up dirt. Sounds great, right? Not all surfactants are created equal, however, and two of them are particularly nasty. **Sodium lauryl sulfate (SLS)** and **dextran sodium sulfate (DSS)** are notoriously toxic for the gastrointestinal system, creating irritation and inflammation. In fact, in their study of inflammatory bowel disease (IBD), researchers use SLS and DSS to give mice colitis.

Your Liver, the Ringmaster

Of course, environmental exposure is only one piece of your body's total toxic burden. You also must detoxify compounds that come from within, from normal metabolic processes. Spent hormones, inflammatory markers and molecules, metabolites, intermediary compounds, and free radicals all must be detoxified, processed, and excreted.

The liver is the ringmaster in the circus of detoxification. It acts in a highly organized, efficient, and intelligent manner. Everything that you take in from the GI tract, everything you drink, breath, snort, or absorb through your skin ends up in the blood. The blood is scanned by the liver, and all of the particles the blood contains are examined. The liver filters almost 1.5 liters (0.4 gallons) of blood per minute—no small feat.

The liver will remove or render safe and let pass back into circulation every single molecule it comes across. It will send many substances—particularly spent hormones and bile—to the large intestine, to be pooped out. It will send some compounds to the lungs to be breathed out, to the kidneys to be peed out, to the skin to be released. For the liver to render a molecule safe it requires many vitamins, minerals, and other compounds. The liver uses the nutrients as helpers, compounds that are required by the body to catalyze the biochemical reactions that render harmful compounds safe.

The waste molecules that the liver packages and ships off to the large intestine have to be pooped out in order to leave the body. If you're not having regular bowel movements, it means waste compounds are staying put in the large intestine. The large intestine has a blood supply, and all that waste gets absorbed right back into the blood supply if things aren't moving along.

Ripple Effects of Not Pooping

It might not sound very important, but consider this: Let's say you eat whole-wheat toast every day for breakfast. You don't know it yet, but that toast is the reason you are constipated. Because you are constipated, you are not pooping out all of the spent estrogens that your liver has already metabolized, packaged, and sent to your colon. As your stool sits in the large intestine, those waste hormones are reabsorbed into your blood.

Remember, anything that gets into your blood gets into your liver. Consequently, your liver has a full schedule dealing with the everyday load of metabolic products and environmental compounds that are present in your blood. Your liver has already dealt once with the estrogen you have just reabsorbed, and now it has to deal with it again in addition to the usual daily load. This doubling up of estrogen—from the day before, plus what is reabsorbed, if it is not pooped out, increases the estrogenic burden on the body, because the estrogens simply are not leaving.

Acne, fibrocystic breast change, premenstrual syndrome (PMS), headaches, brain fog, and a blunted ability to burn fat—particularly in the hips and thighs—are consequences of high estrogen. So, you go to the dermatologist for your skin, the gynecologist for your PMS and painful breasts, and the neurologist for your headaches. They will likely prescribe steroids, antibiotics, birth control pills, muscle relaxers, benzodiazepines, or perhaps a stimulant—when all you have to do to solve these problems is poop!

Perhaps you mention to your doctor that you don't go to the bathroom every day. She may suggest fiber, more water, a laxative, or perhaps even a probiotic, if she's savvy. These methods may work for a while, but ultimately they won't address the WHY of your constipation and increased estrogenic burden—the toast. The Gut Restoration Program in this book (see page 59) will give you the tools to find solutions in your everyday life to problems like this.

The Impact of Hormones on the Digestive System

Your gastrointestinal system makes several hormones and interacts with virtually all other hormones in the body. Hormones are messenger molecules, sent like e-mails to deliver instructions all over the body. Collectively, the hormonal system is known as the endocrine system.

Insulin is a famous hormone made by the pancreas. Your blood sugar is affected by insulin, along with another pancreatic hormone, glucagon. Irritability or lightheadedness when you skip meals, feeling sleepy after meals, and ravenous or low appetite are all signs of blood-sugar imbalance—a situation that can be greatly helped by improving the function of the gastrointestinal tract through the Gut Restoration Program (see page 59). Diabetes is the pathological manifestation of blood sugar gone awry and insulin resistance. Insulin resistance occurs over time when high blood sugar (typically from a high-carbohydrate, low-nutrient diet) elevates insulin to the point at which the body can no longer hear its "message." It is like the boy who cried wolf—your cells have heard it so many times, they are no longer interested in heeding the message.

Leptin, another hormone, plays a key role in regulating energy intake and expenditure, including appetite and metabolism. Acting like the gas gauge in your car, it lets you know when you have had enough to eat. When leptin is high, you feel satisfied and full. Like insulin, it is possible to become resistant to leptin. People with leptin resistance never feel like they can eat enough, even if they are overweight. The Gut Restoration Program acts like a hormonal reset button and helps balance these hormones.

✳

There are a number of other hormones made in the gastrointestinal system for digestive processes. Some of the more important ones are outlined in the following table.

GASTROINTESTINAL HORMONES

Hormone	Function	Released When . . .
Cholecystokinin (CCK)	Slows emptying of the stomach after a meal; ignites digestive capacity by signaling the release of digestive enzymes and bile; increases movement in the colon; promotes a feeling of satisfaction.	You eat a meal with protein and fat.
Gastrin	Fires up stomach-acid production and the release of digestive enzymes.	Protein, caffeine, or alcohol is consumed.
Ghrelin	This is the hormone that gets your belly growling. It makes you feel hungry and gets you thinking about your next meal. Ghrelin also helps repair the intestine.	You have gone without eating for a while, or if you are tired or stressed.

Hormone	Function	Released When . . .
Glucagon-like peptide (GLP-1) and Gastric inhibitory peptide (GIP)	Helps insulin release.	You eat sugar and fat.
Motilin	Helps get things moving! Assists with stomach emptying and movement of the intestines.	Digestive enzymes, bile, and acid are released.
Peptide YY (PYY)	Reduces appetite.	You eat a meal.
Secretin	Releases enzymes, insulin, and sodium bicarbonate.	Acid is sensed in the small intestine.

CHAPTER 3

The Digestive Players

Food makes a long march through your body with the help of many different organs, hormones, digestive factors, and other support. In this chapter, you'll get to know all the characters in your gastrointestinal system and the roles they play, how digestion is supposed to happen under ideal circumstances, and what can go wrong along the way.

The Brain

Digestion starts with anticipation and a thought.

As soon as you begin to see, smell, taste, touch, or think about food—before it even gets to your mouth—your brain begins to communicate with your body in preparation for the incoming meal: Your salivary glands begin to produce saliva; your stomach starts to produce acids and enzymes; your liver increases bile production; and your gallbladder gets ready to release bile. Hormones are released that orchestrate the coordination of digestive "juices" and actions; blood flow is diverted away from your limbs and toward your organs; and you may even have a change in heart or respiratory rate. You are now primed to enjoy your food.

The Mouth

It's hard to have a conversation about digestion without the mouth, right? Included in the mouth are the lips, teeth, tongue, and salivary glands. Saliva is used to soften and lubricate food and to introduce the very first digestive enzymes in the digestive process: amylase and lipase. Amylase begins to break down starch upon contact.

Saliva buffers your food, helps you to swallow, contains clotting factors, and helps protect the teeth and the inside of the mouth. Saliva helps us to absorb nitrates from green leafy veggies. Nitrates are often maligned in mainstream media, but you actually need them for great cardiovascular function. Bacteria on your tongue convert these nitrates into nitrites, which are then incorporated into the nitric-oxide (NO) cycle. NO helps keep the lining of blood vessels healthy, helps lower blood pressure, and reduces inflammation.

The teeth help grind and crush up food, turning it into a paste. Not chewing is frequently overlooked as a cause of gas and bloating. When you eat too fast and don't chew, you inadvertently end up introducing a lot of air into the system and swallowing big chunks of food. Ever notice when you are wolfing down lunch while standing up it doesn't seem to sit quite as well on your stomach? The same sort of thing can happen as you try to avoid chewing because of tooth pain.

Food needs to be broken down into its basic compounds. When you don't chew your food well, more pressure is put on the stomach to break down the food into tiny particles. This delays gastric emptying (the rate at which food leaves the stomach), which then in turn can cause gas, bloating, and fermentation of food. When food is not fully broken down, and larger food particles hit the small intestine, it revolts, causing gas, bloating, and cramping. If this goes on long enough, leaky gut can begin.

✳

Common conditions that are associated with the mouth include apthous ulcers (canker sores), Sjogren's syndrome (an autoimmune condition that causes dry mouth and dry eyes), and halitosis (bad breath).

The Esophagus

The esophagus is the muscular tube that connects the mouth to the stomach. It has two sphincters—the upper esophageal sphincter (UES) and the lower esophageal sphincter (LES). When you swallow, food passes through the UES—the last voluntary digestive action you'll make until you are ready to go to the bathroom.

It takes about 6 seconds for the food to pass through the esophagus and into your stomach, a bit more if the food is dry. When food reaches the bottom of the esophagus, the LES opens like a trapdoor and lets the food plop into your stomach.

The LES is designed to let food into the stomach and keep acid and food con-
its from splashing back up and creating symptoms of heartburn or gastroesoph-
al reflux disease (GERD).

There are many theories about the cause of heartburn. In the vast majority of
es, it is not due, in fact, to excessive acid; rather it is a matter of acid being in
wrong place. Unless you are swallowing food, the LES is supposed to remain
itly closed. However, there are a number of substances that can make the LES
ep open when it is not supposed to, contributing to or exacerbating symptoms
or heartburn. Common culprits are coffee, tea, alcohol, milk, nicotine, orange
juice, spicy foods, mint, onion, anticholinergic drugs, progesterone, calcium-
channel blockers, and diazepam. Consumption of any of these substances can lead
to heartburn or can worsen it.

There is a theory in integrative and functional medical circles that *low* stomach acid also causes the LES to creep open and create heartburn, evidenced
by the resolution of symptoms with the stimulation of stomach acid or HCl
supplementation.

✳

Common conditions that are associated with the esophagus are GERD, heartburn, hiatal hernia (in which part of the stomach herniates, or pushes, through
the diaphragm), eosinophilic esophagitis (EE: in which the esophagus has lots of
eosinophils—a type of immune cell—present, causing irritation and inflammation of the esophagus), Barrett's esophagus (a very specific type of damage done to
the cells of the esophagus, often from repeated exposure to stomach acid or smok-
ing), and achalasia (difficulty swallowing).

The Stomach

What an unsung hero the stomach is! Though the stomach is thought of as a
receptacle or holding depot for food, it is oh-so-much more than that. It is a sac
made of multiple layers of muscles connected to the esophagus and the first part
of the small intestine, the duodenum.

In adults, the stomach is about 10 inches long and can expand to hold 2–3
liters (0.5–0.8 gallons) of food, although one liter (0.26 gallons) will feel a lot more

comfortable. Food typically stays in the stomach for 2–4 hours. The more fiber and fat in the stomach, the longer it will stay there. Aspirin, alcohol, and water are the only substances that get absorbed into the body directly from the stomach. This is part of the reason why you feel the effects of alcohol so much faster if you haven't eaten anything.

The stomach acts like the food blender of the body, crushing, churning, and grinding food down into a soupy concoction known as **chyme**.

The stomach is also the meeting place for bile, digestive enzymes, and stomach acid.

Your stomach is dotted with millions of cells known as parietal cells that are responsible for making hydrochloric acid (HCl). Hydrochloric acid has a pH of 1–2, while the pH of the rest of the body is around 7. The amount of cellular energy required to produce this precious substance is enormous!

HCl packs such a corrosive punch that you don't want it touching any tender parts of your body. Because it is so corrosive, specialized cells in the stomach secrete a thick mucous coating as a barrier to protect the lining of your stomach from HCl. A defect in this lining is called an ulcer.

HCl helps break down proteins, turn on enzymes that further promote digestion, and kill pathogenic bacteria such as harmful *E. coli*, *Campylobacter*, staph and strep, yeast, or any other substance that may have come along with the food you swallowed. HCl is also crucial for maintaining proper bacterial balance in the large intestine and reducing the incidence of yeast infection and urinary-tract infection (UTI).

The stomach, along with the pancreas, produces digestive enzymes. The stomach is also responsible for releasing certain hormones. Ghrelin is a hormone that stimulates hunger—it gets your stomach growlin'—and is mostly made and released by the stomach. The stomach also produces gastrin, a hormone that stimulates the release of enzymes, HCl, intrinsic factor, and other hormones. Additionally, the stomach makes pepsinogen, which turns into pepsin (one of the main enzymes responsible for protein digestion), when it is exposed to HCl. Motilin, another hormone made in the intestine, is responsible for motility (movement) of the intestines and helps regulate the rate at which the stomach empties its contents into the small intestine. (See pages 13–14 for a chart of common gastrointestinal hormones.)

The same cells that make stomach acid—parietal cells—also make a very important substance known as intrinsic factor. Intrinsic factor is crucial for the absorption of vitamin B12. In order for B12 to be absorbed, intrinsic factor must bind to it. When you take acid-blocking drugs that decrease the function of your parietal cells, you are also reducing the production of intrinsic factor and increasing the risk of vitamin B12 deficiency.

In addition to acid-blocking drugs that decrease the functioning of your parietal cells, as you get older, their activity can also decrease naturally. It requires a gigantic effort to produce such a low-pH commodity as stomach acid, and with aging, chronic stress, and poor diet, natural production tapers off, along with levels of intrinsic factor, and the stomach's ability to produce a nice, thick protective mucous coating. By completing the Gut Restoration Program (see page 59), you can freshen the function of your stomach.

✳

Common conditions associated with the stomach are dyspepsia, indigestion, gas, bloating, ulcer, gastritis, hypochlorhydria (low stomach acid), and pernicious anemia (anemia from low vitamin B12).

The Pancreas

The pancreas is nestled in the loop of the first part of the small intestine, the duodenum, and is connected to it by a little duct. The pancreas helps finish what the teeth and stomach have started—the breakdown of big food molecules into very small particles that can be absorbed by the small intestine.

The pancreas is interesting because it serves a variety of roles. It is an endocrine organ, secreting the hormones insulin and glucagon. These hormones are responsible for blood-sugar control, which in turn affects the entire body, including digestive function.

Insulin and glucagon work as a team. When you eat something that causes your blood sugar to rise, insulin is released in order to guide sugar into the cells—feeding them—and thus lowering the amount of sugar in the blood. When blood sugar is low, glucagon is released in order to stimulate the breakdown of glycogen (stored sugar) in the liver and its release into the blood—raising blood sugar. So, the job of insulin is to lower blood sugar after you eat, and the job of glucagon is to raise blood sugar if you have gone too long without eating.

The second role of the pancreas is to make enzymes and other compounds that help break down food molecules and deliver them into the gastrointestinal tract. Lipase and colipase are enzymes that split fat molecules into fatty acids. Amylase (also found in the saliva) breaks up carbohydrate molecules, and the enzymes trypsin, chymotrypsin, elastase, and carboxypeptidase break down proteins into their constituent amino acids. The pancreas even helps break down the deoxyribonucleic acid (DNA) and ribonucleic acid (RNA) of the food you eat with the enzymes deoxyribonuclease and ribonuclease.

As chyme moves from the stomach into the intestine, it has a very low pH after spending all of those hours being mixed with HCl. As it moves out of the stomach and into the duodenum, a hormone called cholecystokinin (CCK) is released. CCK stimulates the pancreas to release an alkaline substance that neutralizes the acidic chyme for the rest of its journey down the GI tract. CCK also stimulates the gallbladder to contract and a host of digestive enzymes to be released in addition to helping you feel full and satisfied.

Low Digestive Fire: Decreased Pancreatic Output

If the pancreas is not able to produce ample amounts of digestive enzymes, problems begin to crop up. When adequate enzymes are not on board, digestion begins to suffer. At first, this may be in the form of irritating but manageable symptoms such as gas, belching, bloating, and undigested food in the stool. Over time, if this is not corrected, it can lead to digestive complaints like leaky gut (when the integrity of the lining of the small intestine is compromised) and food sensitivities. In turn, these can lead to malabsorption of nutrients, which worsens pancreatic enzyme output. This low pancreatic output of enzymes is loosely termed **pancreatic insufficiency** and will reduce digestive fire (the body's ability to break down fat and carbohydrates with the help of acid, bile, and enzymes). Pancreatic insufficiency can be the result of aging, chronic stress, malabsorption of nutrients, malnutrition, food sensitivities, and chronic inflammation. There are also links between pancreatic insufficiency, osteoporosis, and diabetes.

✳

Common conditions associated with the pancreas are pancreatic insufficiency, pancreatitis (acute or chronic inflammation of the pancreas), and type 1 diabetes (DM1), an autoimmune condition in which the immune cells destroy the parts of the pancreas that make insulin, making insulin supplementation crucial for survival. Type 2 diabetes (DM2) is a lifestyle disease in which insulin sensitivity is lost as a result of chronically high blood-sugar and insulin levels. DM2 can thus be cured by diet and lifestyle interventions, although often insulin and other medications are used to control blood sugar.

The Liver

The liver, one of the most complex organs in the body, performs hundreds and hundreds of functions for you every minute. Your liver is one of the most active and dynamic organs, and a good thing, too, because it has so much to do. There are more than 2,000 enzyme systems present in your liver that execute more than 500 functions per minute and manufacture almost 15,000 compounds for your body. That is no small feat, and how much time do you spend each day thanking your liver?

Without your liver, you would die in about 6 hours—not a particularly pleasant thought. But take heart—the liver is tough and hardy: it can lose 70 percent of its function without this stress showing up in a blood test, and it has the ability to regenerate itself.

The liver sits under the ribs on your right side and usually weights about 1.8– 2.7 kilograms (4–5 pounds), taking up a fair amount of space in the abdomen.

All things that are eaten, absorbed, or breathed into your body end up in the liver. The liver's job is to continually filter blood every day—more than 2,000 liters (528 gallons) of blood in one day! That is your entire volume of blood, more than 500 times. Busy indeed!

While the liver is filtering your blood, it will change, metabolize, store, excrete, or detoxify the compounds it comes across. The liver is selfless—if it does not have the ability to detoxify or metabolize a particular compound, it will store it locally inside itself.

The liver changes nutrients into a usable form that can be utilized by your cells; it filters out cholesterol and lipoproteins; removes spent hormones, metabolic products and inflammatory molecules; and packages them up and ships them off to the large intestine, where, hopefully, you poop them out.

When you don't poop out these compounds, they sit in the large intestine and are absorbed back into the bloodstream. Eventually they return to the liver, where they'd been dealt with earlier. Now the liver, busy with today's "junk," has to deal with a backlog of compounds—yesterday's and maybe the day before that too. In this way, you can think of it as if the bowel is constipated, the liver is constipated too.

Bile Basics

Another major job of the liver is the production of bile. Bile is a huge piece of the body's digestive capacity. It helps emulsify and break up fats, just like soap would. Bile helps increase the surface area of fats and spreads them out so that the digestive enzymes have greater access to them and thus split them up better.

Most fats need to be broken down this way so they can be absorbed, assimilated, and incorporated into things such as cellular membranes and hormones. When you have an oily or greasy-looking stool, it is a clear sign you are not absorbing fats.

Made by the liver, bile is composed of bile salts, cholesterol, and lecithin. Yes, cholesterol performs a vital function for the body by contributing to its digestive fire! After bile is made, the liver shuttles it into the bile storage unit: the gallbladder.

The body would not leave a crucial organ such as the liver unprotected, and as such, the liver is rich in immune cells. Kupffer cells are special immune cells that live in the liver and pull bacteria and other compounds from the blood.

The function of the liver can be impaired—though it would never complain—when you are constipated. Although infection and inflammation can disrupt liver function, the liver is very tough and durable overall.

✳

Common conditions associated with the liver are bile insufficiency, hepatitis (inflammation of the liver), cirrhosis (when normal liver tissue is replaced by fibrotic scar tissue), jaundice (often from liver disease), a yellowish pigmentation of the skin and eyes as a result of the liver's inability to clear bilirubin, and NASH (nonalcoholic steatohepatitis, or fatty liver). Alcoholism takes its toll on the liver.

The Gallbladder

Nestled under the liver is a small, pouchlike sac called the gallbladder. Its job is to hold bile, produced by the liver, until it gets the signal to contract and empty its contents into the waiting digestive system to help with the breakdown of fats, cholesterol, and fat-soluble vitamins.

When you eat a meal that contains fat, your body releases a hormone called cholecystokinin (CCK). It signals your gallbladder to squeeze. Remember that this is the same hormone that signals your pancreas to propel enzymes and alkaline substances into the duodenum (the first part of the small intestine)—the first stop chyme makes after it has left your stomach.

Oh No, It's Gallstones!

Dietary factors, particularly fiber and water, are crucial for optimal gallbladder function. The gallbladder is a humble servant of the rest of the GI system. Dysfunctional hormonal signaling arising from a low-fiber diet and impaired gallbladder contraction will inevitably lead to gallbladder "sludge." As bile becomes more and more concentrated and immobile, gallstones develop.

The risk factors for gallstones, the most common problem associated with the gallbladder, include a low-fiber diet and being female, Caucasian, and of childbearing age. Gallbladder removal is one of the most common elective surgeries on the block. In fact, if we took all of the gallstones that have been surgically removed and stacked them in a big pile, they'd reach the moon! This should be excellent motivation to have that salad for lunch.

Here are a few steps to take in order to avoid gallbladder problems—and surgery:

- Incorporate bitter foods into your diet such as dandelion, frisée, endive, and other bitter greens. Artichoke, lemon, and black radish all help with proper bile flow.
- Vitamin C has been shown to reduce gallstone formation. Take 1 gram twice daily.
- Consider decreasing your coffee intake, which can lead to gallbladder attacks.
- After you complete the Gut Restoration Program (see page 59), stay on digestive enzymes for the long term. They will help your body appropriately break down fats and put less stress on your gallbladder.
- Aim for 40 grams of fiber in your diet, every day.
- Take phosphatidylcholine (PC). PC helps make bile more smooth and fluid and less sludgelike, decreasing the formation of stones. Take 100 milligrams two to three times daily.

The Small Intestine

The small intestine is arguably one of the least sexy organs around, but what an interesting and vital role it plays in digestion and your overall well-being. The small intestine is where the vast amount of your nutrition is absorbed, and it is the interface between nutrition and the immune system. All of this action (the interplay of food and the small intestine, interacting with the lining of the small intestine and the immune system) means that if food sensitivities develop, and all of the subsequent inflammation and dysfunctional immune response arise, they do so on the stage of the small intestine.

It turns out that the small intestine isn't very small at all. If you uncoiled all of its many loops, it would stretch about 4.5–6 meters (15–20 feet). It has three parts: the duodenum, the jejunum, and the ileum, which is connected to the large intestine. Anatomically, the three parts are quite similar, but different nutrients are absorbed in each segment.

Calcium, iron, sulfur compounds, magnesium, manganese, zinc, and copper are absorbed in the duodenum. Sugars, including sucrose and other monosaccharides such as glucose, fructose, and galactose, are also absorbed here. Fatty acids (both short and long chain) and the fat-soluble vitamins A, D, and E are taken up in the duodenum and so are vitamins B1, B2, B6, C, and folate.

The **jejunum**, sandwiched between the duodenum and the ileum, also absorbs sugars. Sucrose, lactose, and maltose are taken up in the jejunum. Proteins and amino acids are primarily absorbed in the jejunum, along with several water-soluble vitamins such as vitamins B1, B2, B5, and folic acid.

The **ileum**, the final segment of the small intestine, absorbs cholesterol, bile salts, and vitamin B12.

The Gut Mucosa

The lining of the small intestine goes by a few different names. It is commonly called the gut mucosa and also the brush border or the gut epithelium.

The gut mucosa is completely lined with structures called villi and microvilli. These fingerlike projections help add surface area to the small intestine and increase its absorptive capacity. We've noted that the small intestine is 4.5–6 meters (15–20 feet) long. If you were to completely uncoil and unfold the small intestine and all of its villi and microvilli, it would cover a tennis court! The many thousands of these structures, all folded upon each other, give the small intestine its enormous absorptive capacity. All of the magic happens at the brush border where the nutrition you have consumed and (hopefully) digested and broken down is absorbed into your bloodstream and where harmful materials, bacteria, and yeasts are kept out.

Villi, Microvilli, and Crypts

In addition to greatly increasing the surface area of the small intestine, villi deliver the goods they've absorbed into the blood, block out harmful toxins, and also produce a small amount of enzymes to aid in the breakdown process.

In between the villi and microvilli are crypts, which are like the valleys between mountains, and their job is to continually replace the cells that line the villi. Every day, billions of cells are replaced, but if the villi or the lining of the intestine is inflamed or damaged, those new cells can't work their way to where they need to be. In this case, the crypts become swollen, absorption is hindered, and the small intestine is not as well able to keep the bad stuff out and let the good stuff in.

So much happens at the brush border, and yet it is only one cell-layer thick. That's right. Just one cell layer separates your food, and everything inside your intestine, from your internal environment.

The immune system lies below the brush border. About two-thirds of the immune system resides in the gut.

Unlike the large intestine, which hosts an entire colony of bacteria, the small intestine is largely sterile and devoid of bacteria and other organisms.

The cells that line the small intestine stand very tightly next to one another, like a line of soldiers standing shoulder to shoulder. In fact, they stand so tightly together that there is a structure used to describe it—**tight junction**. These tight junctions are very important for the integrity of the gut because they don't let foreign particles pass through into the bloodstream. An additional structure—a **desmosome**—buttons the cells together. Chronic stress, certain foods, medications, and other environmental toxins can unbutton these desmosomes and weaken the tight junctions, compromising the integrity of the gut wall.

The lining of the small intestine can become compromised from poor nutrition, medications, chronic stress, toxic chemicals from the environment, and aging. When the desmosomes are unbuttoned and tight junctions are not so tight, the immune system has a direct line to food particles found in the lumen of the small intestine—they get to bypass the protective cell layer and the process of absorption through the villi. The immune system then begins to make antibodies against the very food you are eating and generates an inflammatory response.

Leaky Gut

As the immune cells are making antibodies, they also make other compounds to attract more immune cells to the area. They call for backup, and other immune cells arrive. These cells begin making antibodies and inflammatory compounds too. This sets off a cascade of inflammation. Inflammatory compounds released by the immune cells keep the tight junctions open—the immune system has something to attack now—and propel the body forward into a cycle of gut permeability, immune dysfunction, **antibody** production, and exaggerated inflammatory response. It's like a fishing net with holes in it that allow big fish to escape. The fish band together with their buddies and tear the net apart and make a big mess in the water.

This describes the common catchphrase **leaky gut** (in which the lining of the small intestine is overpermeable and overinflamed). With leaky gut, you may notice that you are accumulating food sensitivities and that the foods you used to be able to eat are now giving you problems. Symptoms of abdominal pain, mucous in the stool, bloating an hour after meals, fatigue, headaches, skin conditions, joint pain, nasal congestion, constipation, and diarrhea can all point to leaky gut.

It is possible to test for leaky gut (the lactulose-mannitol test), but the test has a high rate of false negatives, missing a lot of cases of leaky gut. A cornerstone of the Gut Restoration Program is healing the lining of the small intestine and fixing leaky gut. (See page 89.)

If inflammation goes on long enough, absorption can become compromised. The villi can become irritated, blunted, or destroyed by the immune system, impairing absorptive capacity further.

※

Common conditions that are associated with the small intestine are irritable bowel syndrome (IBS); inflammatory bowel disease (IBD) such as Crohn's; microscopic colitis; lymphogenous colitis; Celiac disease (an autoimmune condition in which the immune system destroys the lining of the small intestine upon exposure to **gluten**); intestinal hyperpermeability (leaky gut); small intestine bacterial overgrowth (SIBO, in which beneficial bacteria—which belong in the large intestine—creep up into the small intestine.), and parasitic infection.

The Large Intestine

The passage of food through the large intestine marks the last leg of its journey through the gastrointestinal tract. The large intestine performs a few crucial functions and houses a very important piece of the gastrointesinal system—beneficial bacteria.

The large intestine connects with the small intestine at a juncture called the ileocecal valve. In most people, the valve is by the right hip. Those who are chronically constipated will often ache here.

The large intestine, also known as the colon, is 0.9–1.5 meters (3–5 feet) long and is divided into three parts: ascending, transverse, and descending.

The Appendix

The appendix is a small fingerlike projection that sticks out of the first part of the colon. Once thought of as an organ from the past with no modern function, it is now understood that the appendix plays a vital role in fetal and early childhood development and the maturation of the immune system. The appendix is rich with lymphatic tissue. Poor nutrition, lacking in fiber and rich in refined flours and sugars, can predispose your appendix to become inflamed and necrotic and then rupture. This is known as appendicitis.

The Efficient Colon

The main job of the colon is to absorb water and any remaining nutrients from the chyme, thereby making stool. Roughly two-thirds of stool is water and undigested food and fiber products. The remaining one-third is made up of bacterial cells, both alive and dead.

Each day, more than 7.5 liters (2 gallons) of water pass through the colon, most of which come from body fluids rather than what you drink, although you can now see how important it is to stay hydrated. The colon is efficient at getting most of that water back, about 80 percent.

If the body is not able to recover the water because the stool is passing through too quickly, you get diarrhea. If too much water is pulled back because transit time is slow, stools can become hard and dry and difficult to pass, and constipation is the result.

Stool begins to form in the transverse colon and when it is well formed, it moves down into the descending colon. From there it goes to the rectum.

No one likes to talk about their rectum because it's not a very fashionable topic, but it is a good thing to know a few things about this interesting structure.

The rectum collects stool until there is enough to have a bowel movement. The rectum has two special rings of muscle called sphincters that control the movement of your bowels.

One of the features that make sphincters so amazing is their selectivity: When you pass gas, the sphincters only allow gas to pass—not solids and liquids. The internal sphincter opens when it senses enough stool has collected for a bowel movement.

Time to Go

At this point, the GI system signals to your brain that you are ready to go to the bathroom. This is the only time you will have voluntary control over your digestive process since you swallowed, and it is smart to listen to what your body tells you and go when you get the signal, rather than suppress it.

The external sphincter is under your voluntary control, so you can choose a time and place of your liking to defecate. Ideally, you should have a bowel movement one to three times daily. This is what is considered normal. Passing stool should happen without pain or strain. The stool should be well formed and easy to pass, free of undigested food, blood, or mucous. It should not smell foul enough to knock your socks off and should not appear frothy or greasy.

If you ignore the urge for too long, problems can arise—mostly constipation. Sometimes, however, we are not able to control the external sphincter, resulting in fecal incontinence. There are a variety of reasons for this, such as muscular damage or weakness, chronic diarrhea, chronic constipation, parasitic infection, severe food allergies, hemorrhoids, nerve damage, inactivity, etc. The large intestine can begin to create problems for us when there are dysfunctions arising with peristalsis (the rhythmic, muscular contractions that propel food through the digestive tract), such as constipation and diarrhea. These dysfunctions typically arise from chronic and mismanaged stress, an overreliance on laxatives, and ignoring the urge to defecate when it arises.

✳

Common conditions associated with the large intestine are constipation, diarrhea, IBS, ulcerative colitis (UC) and other inflammatory bowel conditions (IBD), colitis, appendicitis, parasitic infection, polyps (a growth in the intestinal wall that is often not cancerous but should be removed), diverticulosis (a weakness in the intestinal wall that causes a little pouch to form), diverticulitis (what happens when the pouch from diverticulosis becomes inflamed), and hemorrhoids (swollen veins that can remain inside or prolapse outside of the rectum).

Diverticular Disease

The large intestine has to be worked out and exercised like any other muscle or organ for it to perform in tip-top shape. Consuming a fiber-rich diet gives your large intestine the workout it needs. It is commonly thought that diverticulosis, a pouching in the wall of the large intestine when tissues become lax, is caused by a low-fiber diet. On the other hand, if you are chronically constipated—in addition to eating a low-fiber diet—lots of pressure has to be exerted on the wall of the large intestine, which thickens it. This increases pressure even more, causing portions of the wall to blow out, causing diverticulitis.

Diverticulitis happens when these pouches become infected and inflamed—and can be quite serious, often requiring antibiotic treatment. Symptoms of a diverticulitis attack are fever, nausea, vomiting, chills, constipation, and cramping and pain on the lower left side of the belly. If you are having a diverticulitis attack, it is important to go to your doctor right away.

Once the infection and inflammation have cleared, the number-one recommendation is to consume a high-fiber diet, aiming for at least 35 grams of fiber daily. Try to include a mix of high-nutrient, high-fiber foods each day, such as: quinoa (1 cooked cup has 5g fiber), artichoke (1 cooked, medium artichoke has 10g fiber), avocado (½ medium avocado has 7g fiber), steamed green beans (1 cup has 4g fiber), sautéed Brussels sprouts (1 cup has 4g fiber), and a medium steamed pear with skin (6g fiber).

To begin, cook all sources of fiber, including veggies, fruit, and non-glutinous grains such as brown rice, quinoa, and millet.

After you have healed, you may begin consuming raw fruits and vegetables, seeds, and nuts. It is a common misconception that all people with diverticular disease should avoid foods such as nuts, seeds, and popcorn. While these foods are not appropriate in the midst of a flare, they will help whip your intestine into shape, when the waters are calm, and reduce the likelihood of another attack.

The Gut Restoration Program (see page 59) will help prevent further flares by improving the tone of the large intestine and by burnishing your population of beneficial bacteria, which will help prevent future infection.

Beneficial Bacteria

Your large intestine holds another wonder: an enormous volume of beneficial bacterial flora that is collectively called the microbiota. They represent trillions of bacterial cells, which in turn represent thousands of different types of bacteria that can be further broken down into thousands upon thousands of unique species. The microbiota—or gut flora—don't get even a fraction of the respect they deserve.

Did you know that only one out of ten cells in your body is "human"? The rest are bacterial! It makes one wonder who is really in charge, and who is supporting whom.

The microbiota get few kudos from us, it's true, since we humans have a general tendency to be disgusted by bacteria, yet these guys perform innumerable, valuable functions. In fact, they have a comparable metabolic capacity as the liver, and we know how busy that organ is! Gut flora act like an organ unto themselves.

Beneficial bacteria help digest proteins and carbohydrates, including lactose, and can even help improve lactose intolerance. The bacteria help "humanize" nutrients, flavonoids, and other phytochemicals—chemicals we ingest from plants—so that they can be used by our cells and become fully incorporated into the body.

Beneficial bacteria also help your body absorb minerals and even help manufacture a few vitamins to boot—vitamins B1, B2, B3, B5, B6, and K. They help balance intestinal pH and quell intestinal inflammation.

Beneficial bacteria speak to your enteric nervous system, the second brain, and help normalize gut motility and peristalsis.

And there are roles that beneficial bacteria play in seemingly far-flung places. Research suggests that microbiota play a role in heart health by affecting levels of triglycerides and cholesterol. They may even help keep your blood pressure low and affect your rate of aging!

A relatively new and very exciting field of research connected to gut flora is their role in metabolic rate and body composition. People who are obese have different types of flora in their gut than their normal-weight counterparts. By normalizing their gut flora, people who are obese are able to optimize their body composition (i.e., not too fat and not too skinny). People who are obese also have higher levels of inflammatory compounds than those who are not obese, and through supplementation of beneficial bacteria and the subsequent optimization of gut flora, this inflammation can be reduced.

Gut flora also help recycle and break down hormones (they actually enjoy snacking on estrogen and progesterone hormones), bile acids, ammonia, and short-chain fatty acids.

The microbiota in your body is a dynamic and shifting force that continuously recolonizes and re-creates itself. The microbiota is greatly affected by the foods you eat and do not eat, your stress and hydration levels, and the medications you take—particularly acid-blocking drugs and antibiotics. These two classes of drugs are harmful to your gut flora and can set the stage for dysfunction in your gut.

In healthy people, it is common to see very low, minute levels of harmful bacteria and yeast as part of their gut flora. The good guys help keep these bad guys (harmful bacteria and yeast) in check, but sometimes the bad guys can get a leg up. For example, when you take antibiotics, which unscrupulously kill the good guys along with their targets, the opportunistic, rapidly growing bad guys can begin to overgrow and take advantage.

Think of the large intestine as a big ol' parking lot. You want the parking spaces taken up by the good guys—your beneficial flora. If you take an antibiotic, eat foods that are not appropriate for you, or are stressed to the max, the good guys can take a hit and their numbers will be reduced. This leaves an opening for fast-growing, just-waiting-for-a-chance bad guys, and the stage is set for dysbiosis (see page 216). And, because beneficial flora are on such tight terms with the immune system, abnormal immune function can be a consequence when the balance of good guys is tipped.

Modern Nutrition and the Downfall of Digestion

OVER THE LAST SEVERAL DECADES, the incidence of digestive disorders has increased at an exponential rate, in tandem with the rising rates of all chronic disease worldwide and particularly in the United States.

A mere generation ago, irritable bowel syndrome (IBS), a syndrome characterized by diarrhea, constipation, or a mixture of both, was practically unheard of. One of the first-ever references to it appeared in the Rocky Mountain Medical Journal in 1950. Today, IBS affects up to 15 percent of the U.S. population, a number that is likely way below current prevalence, as only about a quarter of people with IBS symptoms seek treatment. The implications reach beyond health and the way we feel. Annually, IBS alone accounts for almost $30 billion in direct and indirect medical costs.

Rates of inflammatory bowel disease (IBD), a cluster of diseases characterized by inflammatory changes in the digestive tract, have increased a whopping hundred fold in the last fifty years. IBD is not nearly as common as IBS, but this skyrocketing rise should make us sit up and pay attention. More than 700,000 hospital visits each year are due to IBD. There are about 1.4 million people with IBD in the United States right now, and the cost of their treatment tips $1.7 billion.

It does not stop there. Prevalence of gastroesophageal reflux disease (GERD)—a condition in which stomach acid splashes out of the stomach and into the esophagus, where it does not belong—constipation, and indigestion have markedly increased during this period. All these trends are leaving a stack of bloated medical bills in their wake.

Several medical and public health experts have declared that the current generation will have a shorter lifespan than their parents, a phenomenon that until now was unheard of. This is due to the greater incidence of chronic disease and the onset of chronic disease in younger and younger people. If our kids are not healthy, the population as a whole is not healthy, period.

This begs the obvious question, what is going on here? Why are we sicker than ever? The answer is fairly straightforward but has many layers: in short, it's our lifestyle, people. The way we eat, sleep, and stress, along with environmental factors and the medications we use, all greatly impact our health and the way we feel.

CHAPTER 4

Nutrition and Digestive Health

My, how times have changed! The nutrition landscape shifts continually, like tectonic plates smashing into one other. One day, eggs are evil. The next, they are wonderful. Eat low fat; eat high fat; eat the right fat. Wait, what's the right fat? Go paleo; be a vegan; only consume raw juice; stay away from pork.

The daily onslaught of nutrition advice, fads, and fiction is enough to give anyone whiplash. Sadly, we are living proof of the fallacy of mainstream nutritional advice. Increasing rates of digestive disorders, obesity, and chronic disease speak louder than the smooth marketing speeches of soft drink companies or the chorus of warnings from the scientific community. While you are in the midst of a storm of conflicting nutrition information and advice, it is easy to lose sight of the bigger picture. However, if nutrition can be viewed in a context that makes sense, concrete themes can be woven together, and a clearer picture of what the human body requires will emerge.

Modern Diet, Caveman Genes

Perhaps the best place to look for ideas about how we should eat today is in the past. What did people eat before the agricultural revolution a mere 10,000 years ago, during the Paleolithic period? This may seem like a long time ago, but given our entire evolutionary history it is but a blink of an eye. Over the millennia, our genetics became attuned to a diet rich in vegetables, fiber, and tubers. Protein was eaten when it was available, depending on the day's kill. Fruit consumption was seasonal, and water was the drink of choice after weaning. Paleolithic people were omnivores whose base nutrition consisted of plants, protein and fat.

Fast-forward to the present. Considering our entire history as a species, the types of food common in today's world have been eaten only for a miniscule amount of time. Our genetics have not had nearly enough time to catch up to this radical dietary change. The intake of high carbohydrates, sugar, corn syrup, trans fats, preservatives, additives, dyes, and fake foods is an assault on our Paleolithic genetics.

The vast difference between what our bodies are designed to eat and what we actually eat is a major contributing factor to the astronomical rates of obesity, gastrointestinal complaints, and chronic disease that are in evidence today.

We are coming to the end of an era that began decades ago, when a low-fat, high-carb diet, championed by the media and medical establishments in a well-intentioned but grossly misinformed attempt to reduce heart disease, has resulted in more obesity than ever, along with a much higher incidence of heart disease. Our children are affected, too: they have high rates of obesity and are diagnosed with cardiovascular disease with greater frequency than ever before; gastrointestinal complaints in children have never been more prominent; and rates of disability from chronic disease and psychiatric issues are frankly alarming.

This is not to say that all carbohydrates are inherently evil 100 percent of the time. However, an emphasis on these types—processed, high-glycemic products displace other, health-giving foods that the body requires to function and feel its best.

What Is Missing?

Like software for a computer, food is like a set of instructions that tells the body how to operate. If your body is fueled with high-quality, nutritious food, you feel well. If your body is provisioned with poor-quality food that is devoid of nutrients and loaded with empty calories, you don't feel quite so well.

One of the major pieces missing from the modern diet is fiber. On average, Americans consume 10–20 grams of fiber daily. Twenty grams of fiber, the upper end of the average intake, might look something like this: ⅔ cup of granola with ½ cup of blueberries (5 grams fiber); a turkey sandwich with lettuce and tomato on two slices of whole-grain bread (5 grams fiber); ½ cup of baby carrots with 2 tablespoons of peanut butter (4 grams fiber); ½ cup of brown rice (2 grams fiber); and ½ cup of green peas (4 grams fiber). Paleolithic people ate more than 100 grams daily, ten times the amount of fiber currently consumed. Why is it so important?

To put it in a few words, fiber is a cornerstone of a healthy digestive system. It slows emptying of the stomach and increases feelings of satiety and satisfaction. Fiber acts as a broom, sweeping the intestines and cleaning them out. It promotes regular bowel function and reduces the risk of all major gastrointestinal diseases, including colorectal cancer.

Soluble Fiber

Soluble fiber refers to fiber that dissolves into the blood, helping to reduce cholesterol and remove inflammatory molecules and spent hormones from the body. Fiber decreases the risk of cardiovascular disease and other chronic conditions. Refined grain products have 400 percent less fiber than their whole-grain counterparts, and even that pales in comparison to the amount of relative fiber found in fruits and vegetables. Fresh fruit contains up to twice the amount of fiber than grains, and vegetables have levels of fiber up to eight times higher than grains. Vegetables and fruits also come with lower sugar content than grains and grain products and a higher phytochemical content.

Phytochemicals

Plant chemicals—phytochemicals—are beneficial components found in high amounts in brightly colored vegetables and fruits. The pigments responsible for the rainbow of colors in fruits and vegetables confer antiaging benefits to the body, reduce inflammation, protect genes from damage (and thus chronic illness and cancer), and move the body toward health. When you are busy chowing down on french fries and the latest mocha frappuccino, you are definitely not consuming beneficial plant compounds.

Omega-3 Fatty Acids

The difference between the types and amounts of fats consumed during Paleolithic times and what we consume today is dramatic—10,000 years ago, the ratio between anti-inflammatory omega-3 fatty acids and pro-inflammatory omega-6 fatty acids was close to one-to-one. This balance is important for immune function and healing, cardiovascular function, cell-membrane fluidity, nerve conduction, and many other functions in the body. Today, Americans consume sixteen to forty times the amount of pro-inflammatory omega-6 fats to anti-inflammatory omega-3 fats. Most of these inflammatory fats come from seed and soybean oils found in virtually all processed snack foods, such as crackers and chips, salad dressings, condiments, and even some oil-packed whole foods such as tuna, sardines, sundried tomatoes, and artichoke hearts. Combined with a low relative intake of rich sources of omega-3 fatty acids from fish and fish oils, for example, the ratio remains shockingly skewed. Research suggests that a ratio above four-to-one of inflammatory omega 6 to anti-inflammatory omega-3 increases the risk for all chronic disease.

The superstars of anti-inflammatory fatty acids are eicosapentaenoic acid (EPA) and docosahexaenoic acid (DHA). They are the building blocks the body uses to make the therapeutic anti-inflammatory compounds that can help offset inflammation developed from inappropriate nutrition, stress, and other environmental inputs. Specifically, they can help reduce inflammation in the digestive system. The food group with the highest concentration of naturally occurring EPA and DHA is fatty cold-water ocean fish, including salmon, mackerel, and herring. The only vegetarian sources of EPA and DHA are a few edible algae, such as spirulina and chlorella.

EPA and DHA are a part of cellular membranes, including the cells that line the gastrointestinal tract. Ideally, cell membranes should be stable but flexible, able to go with the flow. Stiff cellular membranes have trouble communicating with other cells and are more likely to have a shorter life than their limber counterparts (an imbalance of omega-3 fatty acids, pro-inflammatory omega-6 acids, and trans fats make them stiff) . . . another example of the direct correlation between what you eat and the health of the cell membranes in your digestive system.

Embedded in the cell membranes are receptors—and their targets—for different signaling molecules and hormones that act very much like a lock and key. When a particular messenger molecule binds to the receptor, it will issue information that the cell will act on. EPA and DHA play roles in receptor activity and also in appropriate cellular signaling. These fatty acids help all aspects of cellular communication. If inadequate amounts are consumed, the entire communication structure of the digestive system and the body is compromised. DHA is a major component of brain and nerve tissue. Just as insulation on a wire helps with the conduction of electricity, these fatty acids coat the nervous tissue and help with messages and signals coming in and out. Overall, they orchestrate communication within the gastrointestinal tract and aid in peristalsis and improve body-wide communication.

Fatty acids EPA and DHA also act as lubricants for the digestive system. So not only do they aid in the movement of food through the intestines, but they also help make the trip easier. This improves the ease of bowel movements.

We Eat Too Much of the Wrong Stuff Too Often

The body has an amazing ability to compensate but can only take so much. After eating inappropriately for a certain amount of time, symptoms will develop, such as gas, bloating, indigestion, nausea, bowel changes, fatigue, headaches, acne, itchiness, mood changes, and blood-sugar swings. If these are compounded by stress, poor sleep, exposure to harmful chemicals, and a laundry list of other bad habits, diseases are going to manifest. There are a handful of foods prevalent today that accelerate this process.

Gluten

Gluten is the protein molecule that is found in wheat, barley, rye, and some other grains (for a complete list, see page 74). Gluten is what holds bread together and confers texture. It gives pasta chewiness and croissants fluffiness.

Gluten is also a much different molecule than it was even forty to fifty years ago, and it has a greater impact on our health now than it did then. In an attempt to make them more protein-dense and nutritive, gluten-containing grains have been bred over the last several decades, to have ever-increasing protein content. By increasing yields of protein per hectare of grain, the industry and the population it feeds get more bang for their buck. An unforeseen consequence of this breeding is a change in the structure of the gluten molecule from its original state. These days, gluten is a fairly large molecule—in fact, it has double the **chromosomes** of its heirloom predecessor—making it harder for your body to break it down.

Most protein molecules are straight and shaped like a pencil, which makes it easy for them to be broken down by digestive enzymes. Gluten, on the other hand, is spiraled and thus does not cleave and break down easily. When large, unbroken molecules hit the small intestine, gas, bloating, and a dysfunctional immune response are the result.

Sometimes gluten is found with other nefarious compounds that aren't optimal for health. Wheat, in particular, contains the mega-starch amylopectin A. This carbohydrate is extremely inflammatory and provocative to the immune system. It also causes large hikes in blood sugar, contributing to blood-sugar dysregulation, insulin resistance, and obesity. This carbohydrate can raise your blood sugar faster than a slice of white bread (artificially low in amylopectin A) or a tablespoon of white sugar.

Gluten has druglike qualities. **Gluteomorphins** are present in partially digested gluten molecules. As they go through your digestive system, these compounds bind to opioid receptors (the same receptors for morphine and heroin) in the gut, making the body addicted and crave them more and more.

An assortment of diseases, signs, and symptoms are associated with gluten. Between one in 100 to one in 140 people have celiac disease, a genetic autoimmune condition in which the immune system destroys the lining of the small intestine upon exposure to gluten. This sets off a cascade of body-wide effects and malnutrition. Malnutrition then leads to several complications associated with celiac disease: anemia, osteopenia (thinning of the bones, the precursor to osteoporosis), infertility, bruising, dental-enamel defects, fatigue, and brain fog.

Another 21 million Americans are thought to have non-celiac gluten sensitivity. These people do not have celiac disease and small intestine destruction but an immune response is elicited with gluten exposure, culminating in a variety of symptoms that span from head to toe. For example, there can be emotional changes, such as anxiety, irritability, and sensitivity from the inflammation of the blood brain barrier and altered neurotransmitter signaling. Headaches and migraines are also common with gluten sensitivity. Inflammation is at the core of Alzheimer's disease, and gluten is a major driver of inflammation. A variety of skin conditions, including acne, eczema, psoriasis, and dermatitis can be improved with gluten elimination.

In addition, gluten sensitivity has been linked to autoimmune conditions, such as rheumatoid arthritis, lupus, MS, IBD, and Hashimoto's thyroiditis, in which the immune system attacks the body's tissues and cells. If the immune system is making antibodies to gluten, it can also begin to make antibodies to your own tissues or friendly bacteria. This phenomenon is called molecular mimicry and explains how gluten is a common thread in autoimmune disease.

Gluten can also trigger leaky gut. Here's how it works: The cells that line the small intestine stand shoulder to shoulder, tightly forming a barrier like a row of soldiers. Between these cells, there are buttons that keep the cells close to one another, a structure called desmosomes. Gluten is able to unbutton these structures and create space between cells. When this happens, white blood cells (part of the immune system) leak into the lumen of the intestine, creating antibodies to the foods it finds there. The immune cells also release signaling molecules called cytokines that call other immune cells to the area and help keep the desmosomes unbuttoned. The result is more inflammation, more immune stimulation, and more antibody production.

Gluten impacts the joints, making them sore and achy. Thyroid disease, fatigue, and all manner of gastrointestinal complaints ranging from cramps, diarrhea, constipation, reflux, colitis, and IBS to IBD can be triggered or exacerbated by gluten. It doesn't matter if the source of gluten is whole, organic, raw, sprouted, or non-GMO grain. Gluten is gluten, and for many people, it is not a friend to the digestive system.

Soy

The way that Americans have bought into soy hook, line, and sinker represents one of the most clever and successful marketing strategies ever. A quick look at the nutrition label of almost any packaged or processed food will tell you that soy has made it into our food supply in a major way. Soy protein, soybean oil, and soy lecithin are ubiquitous ingredients in these foods.

However, soy is not the health panacea it was once cracked up to be, particularly in the area of gastrointestinal health. Soy contains protease and trypsin inhibitors, enzymes that split up protein molecules. So, when you eat soy, you are shutting down protein digestion. If protein molecules are not broken down into their constituent tiny particles, not only is there decreased absorption of amino acids when they hit the small intestine, but also gastric distress starts up. Sound familiar?

Soy also has a number of oligosaccharides—carbohydrates—that are not recognized by the human GI tract. Ignored, they remain unbroken and create gas and bloating as they reach the small intestine. Oligosaccharides also provoke the immune system, generating an inflammatory response and antibody production, which primes the system for leaky gut, food sensitivities, and molecular mimicry.

Phytates are compounds that reduce the absorption of minerals like calcium, iron, magnesium, and zinc. Soy has some of the highest levels of phytates out there. So, overall, consumption of soy reduces the absorption of amino acids, vitamins, and minerals.

Advocates of soy will point to Asian cultures and their historical use of this plant and reduced rates of cancer. This argument is flimsy on multiple levels. First, Asian populations have lower rates of some cancers found in the West and higher rates of other cancers. This population eats fermented soy, not soy sprinkles, soy burgers, soy cheese, and soy bars. Before the use of fermented soy, the plant was used solely as a crop cover to fix nitrogen for plantings of other crops—it was not used as a food source.

Soy is also a known **goitrogen**, a substance that slows down thyroid function. Soy slows the conversion of inactive thyroid hormone to its active form. The thyroid is a major driver of the metabolic rate, and slowing down thyroid function is like pressing the brake pedal on fat burning.

Bottom line? If you are going to eat soy, make sure it is fermented. The fermentation process breaks down indigestible carbohydrates and dissolves the protease and trypsin inhibitors.

Dairy Products

Milk and milk products including cheese, yogurt, ice cream, sour cream, cream cheese, half and half, and cottage cheese are consumed at a breathtaking rate. According to the Food and Drug Administration (FDA), a single American eats about 14 kilograms (31 pounds) of cheese and more than 272 kilograms (600 pounds) of non-cheese dairy products each year. In contrast, 188 kilograms (415 pounds) of veggies, 7 kilograms (16 pounds) of fish, and 33 kilograms (73 pounds) of poultry are consumed. Americans consume 147 kilograms (325 pounds) of flour and cereal products, about half of which are wheat-based. From this perspective, it is easy to see how grain and dairy products displace other important foods in our diet.

Lactose is the sugar found in milk. Up to 40 million Americans have lactose intolerance, a deficiency of lactase, the enzyme that breaks down lactose. Close to 75 percent of African Americans, Mexican Americans, Native Americans, and Jewish populations are lactose intolerant. This rate of prevalence approaches

90 percent in Asian populations (National Digestive Diseases Information Clearinghouse).

If the lactose molecule is not disassembled in the stomach and remains large and intact, it creates gas, bloating, pain, and indigestion by the time it hits the small intestine. By now, it should be clear that this pattern is common to all large unbroken protein and carbohydrate molecules. If you are lactose intolerant, you will feel better if you take enzymes (particularly, lactase) when you eat dairy products.

Casein is a protein that is found in milk and milk products. For some, this protein is a big problem. Like gluten, it can trigger an inflammatory immune response and prompt antibody production, leading to molecular mimicry and the attack of the body's own tissues. In addition to gastrointestinal side effects, consumption of dairy products can cause headaches, skin rashes, fatigue, and acne and predispose one to urinary-tract infections and yeast infections.

As casein is being digested, **caseomorphins**—compounds that bind to the opioid receptors in the gut—are produced and create cravings and addiction, just like gluten. It's no wonder macaroni and cheese and pizza are in everyone's top ten favorite foods. Often, you don't realize how bad these foods are making you feel until you eliminate them for a time.

CHAPTER 5

The Environment, Stress, and Digestive Health

The world we live in largely influences the landscape of our gastrointestinal tract, including the health of the beneficial bacteria that reside in the intestine. In Section 1 the importance of the microbiota and the myriad services they perform were covered in detail (see page 7). Your gut microbiome helps keep bowel movements regular, balances immune system function, and protects against a variety of infections and diseases. As we learn more and more about beneficial bacteria, connections between health of the good bacteria and blood pressure, cholesterol levels, risk for diabetes, and psychiatric disease are being fleshed out. It seems that gut flora play a major part in determining body composition and predisposition to a variety of chronic diseases. Your nutrition and lifestyle, in turn, greatly affect the health of your gut bacteria.

Assault on the Microbiota

In the United States, one in three babies is born via cesarean section (C-section). In the late '90s, rates of C-section began to steeply increase—not just from region to region in the United States, but even from hospital to hospital. Consideration of birth practices is quite important in the conversation about gastrointestinal health. During vaginal delivery, newborn babies are inoculated with beneficial bacteria from the birth canal, a process that kick-starts the development of microbiota—key factors in shaping the immune system and regulating digestive function. In C-section births, this important bacterial initiation is completely bypassed, and the stage is set for health problems later in life. Unless these babies are supplemented with probiotics following delivery, they do not receive a dose of healthy flora. The implications are serious and include increased incidence of asthma, allergy, ear infection, and food sensitivity.

Formula feeding babies compounds the issue. Breast milk is another delivery method of beneficial bacteria and protective immune molecules that help with the development of both the digestive and immune systems. It is well documented in both research and clinical practice that formula-fed babies experience more allergies, gastrointestinal distress, and food sensitivity than breastfed babies; and they grow into adulthood with compromised microbiota.

Gotta Eat a Peck of Dirt

A number of scenarios present themselves that can further compromise beneficial flora and the development of the immune system. For example, as kids grow up, it's important that they eat dirt, crawl around on the floor, and are licked on the face by pets. This helps to strengthen and develop the immune system and keep it balanced. In today's world, most kids are awash in a tidal wave of antibacterial products ranging from soaps and lotions to foams and gels. The drive to oversterilize everything that comes into contact with kids robs them of immune-building prime time. These products (ubiquitous hand sanitizers and "antibacterial" wipes, etc.) alter gut flora and immune function and contribute to a running list of food sensitivities, environmental allergies, and atopic diseases such as asthma and eczema.

Chemical Exposure

About 2.25 trillion kilograms (5 trillion pounds) of industrial chemicals are manufactured annually in the United States, with the addition of 6,000 new chemicals each year. Safety studies for these chemicals are sorely lacking, and it is unknown how they interact with each other in the human body. It is impossible to avoid all chemical exposure, for the very air we breathe, and virtually all processed foods—even orange juice and ground beef—are loaded with chemicals. You can reduce the risks of exposure, however, by using air and water filters and low-volatile organic pollutants (low-VOC) whenever you are doing any building or remodeling. Choose glass or stainless steel containers and products over plastic for anything you eat or drink (as well as for food and water storage) to avoid chemical contamination, and buy organic produce and low-pesticide foods. To find out which produce is safe, use the Environmental Working Group's Dirty Dozen™ and Clean Fifteen™ lists (see page 304 for information).

A multitude of chemicals are directly toxic to the lining of the gastrointestinal system and the gut flora. Many of them are endocrine disruptors, substances that alter hormonal signaling and give rise to infertility, metabolic dysfunction, fat-loss resistance, and a host of other complaints.

What if MTHFR Mutation Is in Your Genes . . . and What the Heck Is It?

Methylenetetrahydrofolate reductase (MTHFR) mutations are genetic defects in one or both copies of the gene that your body uses to turn folic acid into folate. Folate is the "active" form of the nutrient that your body uses for innumerable functions, such as blood-cell formation, DNA synthesis, and cell growth and division, etc.

MTHFR mutations were only recently discovered—along with a large proportion of the world's population that are affected. People who have a mutation in the gene can experience symptoms of constipation, diarrhea, cramping and spasm, autism, heart disease, depression, and other psychiatric and neurological disorders.

Testing is easy—it's just a swab on the inside of your mouth, a blood draw, or a saliva sample. If you have the mutation, your family should be tested as well, because it is genetic. Treatment is simple and boils down to taking folate along with other supportive nutrients every day.

Stress

Stress is a word that is used so often that it almost fails to have significance anymore. It is taken for granted that everyone suffers from it—and yet stress is a significant and often-dismissed contributor to gastrointestinal symptoms. In Section 1, the "fight or flight" and "rest and digest" branches of the nervous system were described as a seesaw, with the two sides continually balancing each other. (See page 9.)

Chronic stress leads to an imbalance in the nervous system, however, when the fight-or-flight side of the seesaw—the one responsible for stress hormone release—becomes dominant, and pushes down the more peaceful side. As a result, digestive function can become impaired. Symptoms such as reflux, spasm, cramping, gas, and bloating begin to crop up even if they were never present before. Many people who suffer from IBS and IBD say that their condition worsens when they are under stress, and countless others report an upset or "nervous" stomach whenever they face a stressful situation or deadline.

The Power of Positivity

Stress is often a matter of perspective. Ten people can view the same incident and have ten different versions of what happened. It is often your own narrative, the story you attach to a situation, person, or event, that causes you to experience the greatest amount of stress, rather than the actual situation or person. For example, if someone ignores you, you may take it to mean that that person doesn't like you, causing you to feel bad, when in reality, the person may simply not have seen you or perhaps was distracted, and his or her behavior had absolutely nothing to do with you. Reframing an event and focusing on its positive aspects allows you to begin changing your perspective about that person or event, and how you feel and think about it. The gift of a lesson is inherent in everything, from minor annoyances to massive disasters; and by looking for these silver linings, the brain can be trained to be more positive.

The field of neuroscience is not new-age nonsense. It has been expanding at a rapid speed over the last twenty years or so, and researchers in the field have shown that the brain works very much like a filter. The things we focus on in our lives and our state of being translate into how we see the world, and everything else is squirreled away into a spam folder in your mind. If you focus on the negative and what is wrong with the world or a situation, person, or event, you tend to see more negative things in the world. The reverse is also true. You become more positive with each genuine example of positivity that you find around you. This focus on the positive is not about being naive or unaware; it's all about becoming less negative.

Research suggests that the more time we spend thinking negative thoughts, the more impaired our brain function becomes and the less able we are to find creative solutions to problems. So, by reducing negativity in our lives, we are better able to deal with life events as they come and figure out what to do next. For example: Imagine you are at a bank. It is Friday morning. You are looking forward to the weekend. Sunlight is streaming through the window and the weather is perfect. There are others in the bank—children and some elderly people. As you are waiting in line, a robber bursts through the front door. In the subsequent commotion, you are shot in the arm. Cops and the ambulance arrive, you are treated and informed that no one else is hurt and the robber is in police custody. How do you react? You might be indignant and upset: "Why did this happen to me? How could this happen to me? I can't believe I've been shot! Of all the banks in town, why did I have to come to this one?" No one could blame you for feeling this way, but does it help you feel any better? Not really. On the other hand, you might have reacted differently: "Thank goodness no one was seriously hurt. I am so glad those children were not shot. It is a good thing that that elderly man in the corner wasn't shot. What a blessing that I was only shot in the arm. What a relief that they have caught the robber." The situation is exactly the same—you have been shot in the arm—yet the inner dialogue is vastly different. The story around the situation is different. In this way, perspective shapes not only how you view the world, but your state of being as well.

Now Is All We Own

We spend so much time fretting over or reminiscing about what we consider better times in the past—or worrying and anticipating the future—that we hardly notice the moment that is right in front of us.

Mindfulness is a technique that brings the attention to the present moment and engages all the senses with what is happening now. There is a pile of research that demonstrates how mindfulness techniques reduce stress and chronic pain, including gastrointestinal pain.

Anyone can improve the ability to bring mindfulness to the daily acts of life by strengthening the mind's ability to focus. The mind in its "normal" state is very busy, constantly jumping from thought to thought, seemingly at random. Taking a few minutes of each day to consciously focus your mind on breathing, in a simple meditation practice, will help you become more conscious of your passing thoughts and make it easier to bring attention to the present moment. Try the following exercise each day:

Daily Sitting Practice for Calming the Mind

Choose a quiet location where there are minimal distractions. Sit comfortably in a chair, in an upright posture, relaxed, but alert. Your eyes may be closed or half open with a soft focus and directed downward at a 45-degree angle. Close your mouth and tuck your chin in slightly, keeping your jaw relaxed. Place your tongue lightly just above the front teeth at the roof of the mouth. Place your hands palm up or down on your knees or thighs. Focus your mind on your breath, and keep it there. It may help your focus to silently repeat the words *in* with the in-breath and *out* with the out breath. Inevitably, your mind will wander. When that happens, just gently bring your attention back to your breath. You will need to do this over and over again. Each time your mind wanders, just notice, without any judgment, that you've gotten distracted and gently bring your attention back to your breath. You may also occasionally feel your posture sagging slightly. If you do, simply return to an upright, but relaxed, position. Do your best to keep your spine erect and your body balanced, but try not to stiffen up. Imagine your spine as a supple young tree trunk and relax the rest of your body against it. To start, practice for 5 minutes at the same time each day. With regular practice, you can extend the sessions to 20 minutes per day.

Full Body Scan for Relaxation

The simple act of bringing your awareness to different parts of your body in a restful posture is deeply relaxing. Regularly practicing systematic body scans will reduce tension in your body and help restore a "stressed-out" digestive system. Make a recording of your own voice slowly reading the following script, pausing briefly as each body part is mentioned, or ask a partner to read it for you in the same manner while you are lying in a comfortable place. You will experience a reduction in stress if you practice the full body scan even three times a week, but doing it daily will elicit the most noticeable results.

Body Scan Script

- Find a comfortable place where you will not be disturbed to lie down for about 20 minutes. If you are on the floor, you may want to place a pillow beneath your knees to alleviate any pressure on your lower back. You may wish to cover yourself with a blanket, as your body temperature will drop throughout the practice. Lie flat on your back, with your legs about hip-width apart and your arms lying by your sides, palms facing upward.

- To begin your body scan, take three to five deep breaths, making a sound or a sigh as you exhale. Feel all the points of contact between your body and the surface you are lying on soften with each breath. Relax your jaw and tongue. Relax your hands.

- Now begin to notice any sounds you may hear. There is no need to try to figure out what they are; just let them pass through your awareness like light passing through a crystal. As you move through this practice, try to let go of "doing" anything in particular.

- Let yourself be totally at rest. There is nothing to actually do; there is no way to get this wrong. Simply allow your mind to touch gently on each part of your body as it is named. If your mind drifts away or you actually fall asleep, that is totally fine—you will still reap the relaxing benefits.

- You'll be moving attention through different parts of your body one at a time. When you tune in to a body part, you may feel something or you may not. Just allow the occurrence of any sensation or experience you notice, including nothing at all.

- Start in the mouth. Bring all of your attention to the mouth. Notice the lips, the inner walls of the mouth, and the hard palate at the top of the mouth. Notice the tongue. Notice the back of the throat. Notice the teeth, the gums. Notice the presence of any sensations in the whole mouth. The whole mouth.

- Notice your nostrils, your entire nose. Be aware of sensation in your nose. Bring awareness to your right eye, notice sensation in your right eye. Your left eye. Now notice sensation in both of your eyes. Notice any sensations between your eyes, on your forehead. Notice any sensation inside your right ear, your right ear. Notice sensation in your left ear. Notice any sensation in both of your ears. The whole face. Feel the whole face. The whole face.

- Notice sensation in your scalp, the back of the head. The whole head. Let yourself feel the whole head. The back of the neck, inside the throat, left collarbone, right collarbone.

- Move your attention down into your left shoulder, armpit, left upper arm, elbow, lower arm. Notice any sensation in your left palm, fingers of the left hand. Notice sensation in your entire left arm and hand. Your whole arm and hand.

- Now, move your attention to your right shoulder, right armpit, upper arm, right elbow, lower arm. Notice any sensation in your right palm, fingers of the right hand. Notice sensation in your entire right arm and hand. Your whole arm and hand.

- Bring your attention to your chest, your solar plexus, your belly, your whole abdomen. Notice any sensations inside, in the middle of your abdomen.

- Notice the whole length of the spine. The whole spine. Notice any sensation in your upper back, middle back, lower back, sacrum. Notice sensation in your entire torso. Your torso. Your whole torso.

- Bring your attention to the bowl of your hips and pelvis, to your buttocks, your left thigh, left knee, left calf, ankle, sole of the foot, toes of the left foot. Notice sensation in the whole of the right leg and foot. Your whole leg and foot.

- Notice your right thigh, knee, right calf, ankle, sole of the foot, toes of the right foot. Notice sensation in the whole of the right leg and foot. Your whole leg and foot.

- Feel both legs. Notice sensations in both of your legs. Both legs.

- Feel your entire body, your entire body. Your whole body. Feel your whole body. Notice any sensation in the back of your body, the back of your body. Notice sensations in the front of your body, the front of your body. Notice the left side of your body, the entire left side. Notice the right side of your body, the whole right side. Bring your awareness to your whole body. The whole body. Be present to any experience you notice. (Pause silently for a minute or two.)

- Now begin to deepen your breath. Notice the points of contact between your body and the surface beneath you. Begin to notice any sounds. Notice the sound of your own breath. Run your tongue around your teeth inside your mouth. Slowly begin to twitch your fingers and toes. Create a gentle, gradual transition for yourself back into awareness of the room in which you are lying. Imagine yourself moving into the next part of your day. When you are ready . . . there is no hurry . . . take as much time as you need . . . gently open your eyes and let your gaze be soft as you continue to lie restfully on your back. Let your eyes close again and roll over onto your left side for a few moments. When you are ready, gently return to a sitting position and rest until you feel ready to stand and move into the rest of your day.

CHAPTER 6

Medications and Digestive Health

Gastrointestinal symptoms top the list of side effects for many classes of medications. In fact, WebMD states that nearly any drug can cause nausea or an upset stomach. It cannot be overstated how profoundly appropriately prescribed drugs can affect normal digestive function and impact the way we feel. This is by no means a call to discontinue the use of medication but to take a hard look at whether pharmaceutical drugs could be contributing to our current state. Are there alternatives to drugs? Is it possible to make lifestyle changes to reduce the need for drug therapy? These questions warrant consideration for those of you whose medications are contributing to or exacerbating your symptoms.

Commonly Prescribed Drugs with Gastrointestinal Side Effects

Prescriptions for gastrointestinal complaints have been skyrocketing in the United States and are among the most common drugs prescribed, topped by the giant classes of psychiatric medications, anti-cholesterol agents, and painkillers. More than 4 billion prescriptions are filled each year. The Centers for Disease Control and Prevention (CDC) asserts that close to 48 percent of Americans are on at least one pharmaceutical drug. With rates this high, it would be a gross oversight not to include them in a discussion about gastrointestinal health.

Nonsteroidal Anti-inflammatories (NSAIDs)

One of the most infamous classes of drugs that manifest gastrointestinal side effects is nonsteroidal anti-inflammatories (NSAIDs) such as aspirin, ibuprofen, and naproxen. Chronic use of NSAIDs irritates the lining of the gastrointestinal system. Ulcers, gastritis, indigestion, and inflammation of the esophagus are common side effects of NSAIDs. Typically, this class of drugs is prescribed for controlling pain and inflammation associated with headaches, menstrual pain, arthritis, and other musculoskeletal complaints.

NSAID use is on the rise, with 70 million prescriptions written annually, along with 30 billion over-the-counter purchases. NSAIDs are considered safe, yet they still account for more than one 100,000 emergency room visits—roughly 40 percent of all drug-related visits—and more than 16,000 deaths per year (equaling the number of people who overdose on painkillers annually). Many of these consequences are preventable. A recent study found that 43 percent of prescription NSAIDs were unnecessary.

Antibiotics

Antibiotics are a commonly prescribed class of drugs with a high rate of gastrointestinal disturbance. These drugs are designed to kill bacteria, and they do a pretty good job of it. Antibiotics are indiscriminate killers, however, and destroy beneficial bacteria in addition to pathogenic bacteria. If the balance of healthy gut bugs is altered, it makes the body more vulnerable to an overgrowth of harmful bacteria and yeast in the long term. This is particularly true if probiotics are not taken concurrently with antibiotics.

Indeed, major side effects of antibiotic use are stomach pain, diarrhea, and infection with *Clostridium difficile* (a type of bacterial infection, often following antibiotic therapy, that causes severe diarrhea and roughly a 7 percent death rate). Indeed, many people who suffer from these side effects report a direct link between the onset of their symptoms and taking antibiotics—and the clinical evidence is there. Most of these people are never told by their doctors to take probiotics, which help offset the negative side effects of antibiotics without reducing their efficacy.

Each year, 100 million prescriptions are written for antibiotics. The CDC estimates that half of these prescriptions are inessential. Antibiotics do not work against viruses, yet antibiotics are often prescribed for viral infections that cause coughing, flu, and respiratory infections. Antibiotics have been prescribed for asthma, which has no biological justification unless an asthmatic person gets a bacterial infection. The irresponsible overprescription of antibiotics is the leading cause of the development of "superbugs"—bacteria that are antibiotic resistant. When bad bugs aren't killed by the usual tricks, there are fewer tools to use, and there is a greater likelihood that complications will set in from infection, such as tissue death (necrosis) and sepsis, a life-threatening condition where bacterial infection spreads into the blood. The judicious use of antibiotics, concurrent with the use of probiotics, is essential to minimize side effects, prevent future concerns, and reduce the development of antibiotic-resistant superbugs.

Opiates

Opiates are a class of painkilling drugs that are currently enjoying blockbuster sales. Percocet, Vicodin, and Hydrocodone are examples. Opioid drugs work by greatly reducing nervous system activity and, through this action, are capable of grinding digestion to a halt. Constipation is the number-one side effect of opiates. Many people who take these drugs also have prescriptions for over-the-counter laxatives.

Using laxatives over the long term, however, is not the answer to constipation brought on by the use of opiates, because they compromise the body's ability to regulate bowel function on its own. Overuse sets the stage for laxative dependence, which can be difficult to reverse. Opioids themselves are highly addictive with a high potential for dependency. As such, they should be reserved for extreme cases of pain, for use after a major surgery, for example, or for cancer or end-of-life circumstances. Opioids should not to be prescribed for bumps and bruises—not even broken bones or dental work.

Other Prescription Medications

Acute pancreatitis is a painful condition that can range in severity from abdominal discomfort, nausea, and vomiting to debilitating pain and damage to internal organs that requires hospitalization and puts one at risk for death. Pain is often in the upper abdomen and radiates to the back, and can be accompanied by fever, chills, loss of appetite, shortness of breath, and shocklike symptoms. There are many causes for acute pancreatitis, one of the most prominent of which is prescription medications.

A survey in 2003 revealed that furosemide (a diuretic), corticosteroids, azathioprine (an immune suppressant), and sodium valproate (used for epilepsy and anorexia) are the drugs most likely to induce acute pancreatitis.

Alendronate is a bisphosphonate drug prescribed for osteoporosis. The debate concerning true efficacy of this class of drugs rages on. A major side effect of this widely prescribed drug is ulceration of the esophagus.

It is even possible that the side effects of certain drugs are exact mimics of certain digestive disorders! Benicar (olmesartan), a medication used for blood pressure, generates celiac disease–like illness. Between 2008 and 2011, fourteen Benicar users were hospitalized for vomiting, weight loss, diarrhea, and intestinal inflammation and destruction, the classic presentation of celiac disease. In fact, the working diagnosis for this group of people was celiac disease. However, they were not getting better with a gluten-free diet, the typical treatment for celiac. Symptoms only regressed when Benicar was discontinued. Although only fourteen were hospitalized, many more experienced symptoms.

Another possible offender is liraglutide. As rates of type 2 diabetes increase, so do the options for drug treatment. Liraglutide is a medication used to reduce blood sugar in diabetics. Nausea, vomiting, and diarrhea are common side effects of liraglutide, which is often used in conjunction with metformin, another medication that helps to lower blood sugar. In turn, metformin depletes vitamin B12, a vitamin crucial for cellular energy.

The Dark Side of Acid-Blocking Drugs

It is a damning commentary about the state of the nation's collective gastrointestinal system that Nexium, "the little purple pill," is in the top three most commonly prescribed medications in the United States. Nexium is available over the counter and generates a staggering amount of money in sales.

Although they are popped like candy, proton pump inhibitors such as Nexium (as well as Prevacid, Prilosec, Omeprazole, and other acid-blocking drugs), are not without significant side effects, because they reduce the amount of acid produced by the cells that line the stomach. Typically, reflux and heartburn are not caused by too much acid but by acid in the wrong place. While reducing acid can help with short-term symptom relief, it can also exacerbate the underlying reasons why reflux is occurring in the first place and create additional gastrointestinal problems.

Acid is required to digest proteins. If these drugs are taken for more than several weeks to months, protein digestion will be compromised. Proteins that aren't fully broken down provoke the immune system and can irritate the lining of the small intestine, generating inflammation that could lead to leaky gut (which occurs when the lining of the small intestine is compromised, allowing food molecules and immune cells to interact and create further inflammation, food sensitivities, and problems with absorption).

The same cells that make stomach acid also make intrinsic factor. Intrinsic factor is a compound that binds to vitamin B12 and makes it readily absorbable by the body. By slowing these cells, intrinsic factor is reduced, and so is the body's ability to absorb vitamin B12. Acid is required for the absorption of other nutrients, including calcium, iron, magnesium, and folate. If long-term use of proton pump inhibitors impair the body's ability to absorb these nutrients, it is possible for nutritional insufficiencies to develop, such as anemia.

Acid also helps maintain appropriate intestinal pH, which reduces infection by yeast, pathogenic bacteria, viruses, and parasites. Proton pump inhibitors and other acid-blocking drugs raise intestinal pH and leave the body more vulnerable to infection. In fact, clinical studies have shown that risk for C. *difficile* infection is doubled for those who take proton pump inhibitors. C. *difficile* causes diarrhea, cramping, and intestinal spasm, and has a fatality rate of about 7 percent and up to 20 percent in some compromised/vulnerable populations. Proton pump inhibitors promote small intestine bacterial overgrowth (SIBO) and make the body more vulnerable to all types of bacterial infection.

A survey of a half a million medical records demonstrated that the use of proton pump inhibitors is associated with an increased risk of community-acquired pneumonia. In hospital settings, use of these medications is linked to antibiotic-resistant bacterial infections.

Acute interstitial nephritis is an irritation of the kidney that can sometimes lead to kidney failure. Proton pump inhibitors are one of the most common classes of drug that trigger nephritis.

In the elder population, long-term use of proton pump inhibitors increases risk of hip fractures and osteoporosis. These drugs impair the absorption of bone-building minerals.

It is possible that proton pump inhibitors have cardiovascular side effects as well. The *Canadian Medical Association Journal* published a six-year-long population study of people who have had a heart attack that linked the use of these drugs to a 27 percent increased risk for a second heart attack. Proton pump inhibitors diminish the antiplatelet benefits of the drug Plavix, which is often prescribed after a heart attack to prevent a second attack.

Astra Zeneca, creators of Nexium, gave the Food and Drug Administration (FDA) data from two studies that showed people taking Nexium were at an increased risk for heart attack and congestive heart failure. The data were provided in 2007, and the FDA at that time did not take action or issue any warning to the public. Late in 2007, the FDA dismissed the data, qualifying the events as related to age or preexisting conditions. Typical of the FDA. Horrendous.

The Gut Restoration Program

As you embark on this journey, the primary objective is for you to feel better. As an added bonus, you will be improving the health and function of your gastrointestinal tract and pulling your immune system back from the autoimmune edge. You will find a questionnaire to help you pinpoint specific areas that may be troubling you (see page 61) and learn exactly how to find out which foods work for your body and which foods don't. This section will walk you step-by-step through a complete Gut Restoration Program that anyone can use and benefit from, no matter what the trouble happens to be. You will also find a complete twenty-eight–day meal plan along with recipes, a supplement schedule, and a bit of troubleshooting to help make the process as seamless as possible.

CHAPTER 7

What to Expect

The goal of the Gut Restoration Program is to reduce common symptoms such as gas, bloating, pain, reflux, and cramping—whether they are isolated symptoms or part of a disease process—by tuning up the gastrointestinal tract. Other objectives are to promote regularity and consistency of bowel movements (no more racing to the bathroom or struggling to go for days on end) and to create an effective immune system, one that is neither too stimulated and attacking tissues of the body nor one that lets viruses, pathogenic bacteria, and other unsavory characters slide by.

Pinpointing Your Symptoms

The purpose of the Gut Restoration Program is to effectively target and heal all major areas of digestive function that contribute to gastrointestinal distress and underpin digestive disorders. The following symptom checklists will help you hone in on areas that may be particularly troublesome for you. By following the Gut Restoration Program (see page 72), all of these areas will be addressed. You will learn how to identify and eliminate food sensitivities; spruce up digestive fire (in order to break down food more effectively); help your beneficial bacteria become more robust; heal the lining of the gastrointestinal tract; and balance stress so that your nervous system does not have a deleterious effect on your digestion and health.

Could the Food You Are Eating Be Making You Sick?

Undiagnosed and unknown food sensitivities play a major role in chronic gastrointestinal (GI) disturbance. Until fairly recently, the idea—that food could impact digestion and health—was broadly dismissed by the conventional medical community. Research is now bearing out what anyone with common sense has always known: not all foods are appropriate for all people. Understanding what foods may make you feel bad arms you with information and insight into your body and how it works.

SIGNS OF FOOD SENSITIVITY

Do you have this symptom?	Yes	No
Gas		
Bloating		
Bloating that gets worse as the day goes on		
Constipation		
Loose stool		
Inability to lose weight		
Pernicious anemia		
Iron-deficiency anemia		
Heart palpitations after eating		
Wheezing after eating		
Acne		
Fatigue		
Brain fog		
Seasonal allergies		
Insomnia		
Anxiety		
Depression		
Thyroid disease		
Sore joints		
Frequent colds		
Fibromyalgia		
Multiple chemical sensitivities		

If you checked yes to ten or more of these symptoms, it is highly likely that you are eating a food that you are sensitive to. As you follow the Gut Restoration Program, you will learn how to identify those foods.

Do You Have Good Digestive Capacity?

The body's ability to break down food is paramount for digestion and health. Adequate stomach acid, enzymes, and bile help achieve this goal. A lack of any one or all of these factors will impair digestion.

SYMPTOMS OF LOW STOMACH ACID

Do you have this symptom?	Yes	No
Low appetite		
Get full quickly while eating		
Food feels like it sits in the stomach		
Nausea		
Nausea with supplements		
Frequent belching; belches may be foul		
Bloating 1–2 hours after meals		
Frequent stomach upset		
Chronic constipation		
History of acid-blocking drugs		
Difficulty digesting meat and other protein-dense foods		
Reflux		
Regurgitation of food		
Undigested food in stool		
Anemia		
Weak, peeling nails		
Rectal itching		
Known food sensitivities		
Sour taste in mouth		
Frequent yeast or UTI infections		
Coughing, particularly at night		

If you have checked the yes box for six or more of these symptoms, low stomach acid may be a problem for you. Over a four-week period, the Gut Restoration Program will rebuild your digestive capacity.

SYMPTOMS OF LOW ENZYME
OUTPUT/PANCREATIC INSUFFICIENCY

Do you have this symptom?	Yes	No
Bloating within 3 hours of eating		
Frequent lower gas		
Undigested food in stool		
Foul-smelling gas and stool		
Tiredness after meals		
Loose stool		
Stool is shiny or light		
Stool has mucous in it		
Cramping		
Constipation		
Fiber-rich foods cause constipation		
More than three bowel movements daily		
Dry skin, hair, and nails		
Reflux		
Trouble gaining weight		

If you have checked the yes box for four or more of these symptoms, low enzyme output may be contributing to your symptoms.

SYMPTOMS OF DYSFUNCTIONAL BILE OUTPUT/LIVER COMPROMISE

Do you have this symptom?	Yes	No
Cannot digest fats well		
Pain after fatty meal		
Bad breath		
Pain under the ribs on the right side (liver)		
Constipation		
Difficulty passing bowel movements		
Stool is light colored		
Stool floats		
Stool is foul smelling		
Blood in the stool		
Stool is painful to pass		
Jaundice/yellow-tinted skin		
Whites of the eyes are yellowish		
Strong body odor		
Gallbladder surgery		
History of gallstones		
Headaches after meals		
Face/body is puffy from water retention		
High cholesterol		
High triglycerides		
Gout		

If you checked yes to more than eight of these symptoms or have had your gallbladder removed, bile function may be compromised.

During the course of the Gut Restoration Program, you will boost your overall digestive capacity by replenishing stomach acid, digestive enzymes, and bile.

Are Your Beneficial Bacteria Happy?

A thrifty bacterial population in the large intestine provides us with many health-giving attributes. When they are not in balance, problems arise.

SYMPTOMS OF DYSBIOSIS
(BACTERIAL IMBALANCE)

Do you have this symptom?	Yes	No
Sugar causes bloating		
Fiber causes bloating		
Carbohydrates cause bloating		
Cannot tolerate probiotic supplements		
Chronic diarrhea		
Belly is distended		
Belly pain		
Frequent infections		
History of antibiotic use		
Diagnosis of IBS		
Restless legs syndrome		
Fibromyalgia		
Using acid-blocking drugs		

If you checked yes to more than five of these symptoms, it is a priority for you to address dysbiosis with the Gut Restoration Program.

Candida

Candida overgrowth can masquerade as a variety of other signs and symptoms. Ideally, if you suspect candida overgrowth, it should be confirmed with stool or blood testing, but this checklist can give you some clues.

SYMPTOMS OF CANDIDA OVERGROWTH

Do you have this symptom?	Yes	No
Chronic vaginal infections		
Chronic urinary-tract infections		
Chronic sinus infections		
Frequent colds		
Toe/fingernail fungus		
Rashes under breasts/in armpits/groin		
Alternating constipation/diarrhea		
Symptoms worsen with sugar		
Symptoms worsen with alcohol		
Symptoms worsen with fermented foods		
Symptoms worsen on rainy or muggy days		
Blood-sugar swings		
Brain fog		
Bloating		
Anxiety		

If you checked yes to more than eight of these symptoms you could have Candida. Testing for confirmation of Candida and other forms of dysbiosis is highly recommended. Testing and treatment options are fully detailed on pages 228–231.

Health of the Lining of the Gastrointestinal Tract

Ensuring the integrity of the lining of your digestive tract is one of the most important things you can do for your digestive health and overall well-being. This lining is the interface between your nutrition, immune system, beneficial bacteria, and body. A problem with the lining of your GI tract has the ability to cause problems throughout your body, like a collapsing house of cards.

SYMPTOMS OF ULCER OR GASTRITIS

Do you have this symptom?	Yes	No
Gnawing pain in the stomach		
Stomach pain relieved within an hour of eating		
Stomach pain relieved by carbonated drinks		
Stomach pain relieved by milk		
Unremitting stomach pain		
Belching		
Bloating		
Ulcer		
Butterflies in stomach		
Symptoms worse when upset		
History of acid-blocking drugs		
History of NSAID use		

If you checked yes to more than eight of these symptoms, you could have an ulcer or gastritis. If you suspect you have an ulcer, it is important to discuss it with your doctor.

Leaky Gut

The lining of the small intestine is like a smart filter, strategically letting some things in—such as broken-down food particles and nutrients—while keeping others out, such as pathogenic and environmental toxins. When this integrity is breached, the smart filter is compromised and bypassed. This creates a host of consequences, including inflammation, abnormal immune response, and food sensitivities that manifest a wide range of symptoms.

SYMPTOMS OF LEAKY GUT (INCREASED INTESTINAL PERMEABILITY)

Do you have this symptom?	Yes	No
Constipation		
Diarrhea		
Belly pain		
Bloating		
Distended belly at the end of the day		
Multiple food sensitivities		
Unable to tolerate foods that were previously well tolerated		
Multiple environmental allergies		
Chemical sensitivities		
Sensitive to smells		
Water retention		
Belly pain		
Chronic fatigue		
Mucous in stool		
Chronic nasal congestion		
Acne		
Eczema		

Do you have this symptom?	Yes	No
Rashes		
Frequent headaches/migraines		
Mood swings		
Symptoms worsen with alcohol		
Use of antibiotics		
Use of NSAIDs		
Diagnosis of celiac disease		
Diagnosis of Crohn's disease		
Diagnosis of ulcerative colitis		
Diagnosis of IBS		
Diagnosis of rheumatoid arthritis		

If you checked yes to more than ten of these symptoms, it is likely that the integrity of your gastrointestinal lining is compromised and contributing to your symptoms. A major tenet of the Gut Restoration Program is healing the lining of your digestive tract.

Goals and Benefits of the Gut Restoration Program

During these next four weeks, you will pull together several interventions that will bolster the health and function of your digestive system: You'll feel more energized and experience sharpened mental clarity; your aches and pains will dissipate; and your skin will clear as a natural result of this process. Along the way, you will learn a lot about what your body needs to work at its best.

The following list summarizes the main goals and benefits of the Gut Restoration Program:

⊚ The first goal of the Gut Restoration Program is to remove any potentially irritating or allergenic foods, substances, and pathogens from your diet. This includes removing allergenic and inflammatory foods that are "big bullies," along with any foods that you know you are sensitive to. In addition, you will be taking stock of your personal-care products as well as the products you use in your home, to determine if any of them are detrimental to your gut health.

If you think you have a yeast overgrowth, a parasite (40 percent of people who have IBS have one), or a bacterial infection, we will show you how to test for and eradicate these infections as well.

◎ Next, probiotics will be used to bolster your beneficial flora and make them more robust. Probiotics help the immune system navigate the terrain of the body and can keep autoimmune reactions at bay. You've probably noticed the recent onslaught of commercials espousing the many benefits of probiotics that are added to yogurt, butter, drinks, or simply taken as a supplement. The media is finally catching up with what integrative and complementary health providers have known for decades.

◎ Third, your digestive ability is going to be increased. Many gastrointestinal conditions can crop up simply because you don't have enough "fire" to break down foods into tiny, digestible particles. This small detail is often overlooked and is frequently the main culprit in the development of gas, bloating, and cramping, as well as a contributing factor in the development of food sensitivity. Supplementing your diet with digestive enzymes helps your body break down foods and gives your body a polite wake-up call that says, "Start making your own enzymes!" In certain cases, supplemental acid or bile may be warranted. In the case of bile supplementation, vegan or bovine products are used as stand-ins for bile in order to help people (who have had their gallbladder removed and are experiencing difficulties eating) increase their ability to break down and thus digest and absorb fats.

◎ The crown jewel of the program is the reparation of the lining of the gastrointestinal system, in particular the lining of the stomach, with its thick mucous layer and assortment of specialized cells; and the epithelial barrier of the small intestine, which is especially vulnerable to injury—once it is compromised, it will need some help to repair itself. The lining of the small intestine is often an unsuspected source of symptoms. Until its integrity is restored, it will continue to sabotage the best diet, probiotics, enzymes, etc. Once you've healed the lining of the small intestine, you can close the door on your tummy troubles. In this program, you will be using a selection of key supplements to cure the sensitive lining of your digestive tract.

Who Can Benefit from the Gut Restoration Program?

By now you are likely beginning to realize the enormous reach that the gastrointestinal system has into other systems of the body and the great impact it has on your well-being and everyday bodily function.

The Gut Restoration Program is very helpful for people struggling with chronic, general GI symptoms that never seem to go away completely. Constipation, diarrhea, indigestion, low appetite, cramping, gas, and bloating are all greatly improved by this tune-up.

The program is also beneficial for those of you who have been diagnosed with conditions such as IBS (irritable bowel syndrome) or IBD (inflammatory bowel disease: Crohn's disease, ulcerative colitis, microscopic colitis, lymphagenous colitis), reflux/GERD, and celiac disease.

Additionally, if you are experiencing symptoms after an event such as travel or infection, this program is for you. If you have multiple sensitivities to foods, chemicals, and perfumes, check it out.

Certain gastrointestinal diseases are autoimmune in nature or have an autoimmune component. Because two-thirds of the immune system resides in the gastrointestinal tract, many autoimmune conditions—not just the ones based in the digestive system—can be improved with the program.

People with multiple sclerosis (MS), lupus, autoimmune thyroid disease (Hashimoto's thyroiditis or Grave's disease), Sjorgren's syndrome (an autoimmune condition in which the body attacks and destroys salivary glands, creating dry mouth), and rheumatoid arthritis (RA) have gone through this program with great results, including fewer symptoms and reduced levels of inflammation and autoantibodies in the blood.

Skin problems such as non-specific rashes, dermatitis, eczema, psoriasis, chronic rashes, seborrhea, dandruff, and acne should clear up after a few weeks on this program. The skin is a mirror for the digestive system, and the program will clean troubles up from the inside out.

Lastly, this program can help you too if you suffer from unremitting and/or unresponsive migraines; a history of headaches; chronic brain fog or decreased brain power; anxiety; depression; chronic yeast infections; chronic urinary-tract infections; chronic sinusitis, or osteoarthritis.

CHAPTER 8

Getting Started on the Gut Restoration Program

As you begin the Gut Restoration Program, keep a few things in mind. First, always listen to your body. Your unique sensitivities trump any list. If you know you are sensitive to an item remove it, even if it is not specified here. Next, it is possible that you may feel tired, foggy, or off in some other way for a few days after starting this program. This is a normal reaction to dietary changes and typically resolves in 72 hours. Know that this program has a set time schedule from beginning to end, and it is not something you are going to be hooked into forever. Lastly, this program is going to help you perform a lot of detective work on your body. You will likely be identifying food sensitivities—and noticing how your body responds to them—in ways that may have slipped your attention before. Collecting this data will help you reach the main objective: feeling better.

The Gut Restoration Program at a Glance

This is a quick reference guide for the Gut Restoration Program. All of these steps are to be done at the same time, for four weeks:

Step 1. Remove irritating foods

- Eliminate gluten, dairy products, soy, nightshade vegetables such as white potatoes, bell peppers (all peppers, except black pepper—the spice), eggplant, tomatoes, beans, legumes, alcohol, sugar, and other sweeteners.
- Utilize the meal plans (see page 96) and list of "powerfoods" (page 97) to incorporate into your diet.

Step 2. Take a probiotic

◉ Take 50–100 billion colony-forming units (CFUs) of probiotic featuring *Lactobacillus* and *Bifidobacteria* strains (see page 84).

Step 3. Boost digestive ability

◉ Take two capsules of plant enzyme digestive formula with meals (see page 86).
◉ If indicated, take 500 milligrams betaine HCl with meals (to see if you would benefit from stomach acid, see page 88).

Step 4. Repair the gut lining

◉ Take a gut-restoring complex of nutrients (see page 90).

Step 5. Lifestyle changes

◉ Establish a bathroom routine (see page 93).
◉ Establish a good sleep routine (see page 94).
◉ Utilize stress-reduction techniques (see pages 49–51, 95, and 190).

Getting Started on the Gut Restoration Program

It's time to dive in! During the program you will be cleaning up your diet, environment, and digestive system in order to elevate your digestive ability, increase the health of your beneficial bacteria, soothe and heal the lining of your digestive tract, and calm and balance your nervous system and the "second brain" that resides in your gut. All of the following steps are to be done concurrently for four weeks. After the four weeks, it will be time to assess your symptoms and either modify your diet or come off the program altogether.

STEP 1. Remove Irritating Foods

◉ The first step in the program is to remove the big bullies—the most irritating foods—from your diet, even if you think you can tolerate them well. Certain foods are inherently inflammatory and can create a dysfunctional immune response. These foods can be directly compromising to the digestive system, and in an already irritated system, they add fuel to the fire—so they have to go. At the end of the program, you can start eating these foods, one at a time, to assess your reaction to them, and at that time you will know for sure whether they are friend or foe.

◎ **Gluten-containing grains.** Wheat, barley, rye, muesli, spelt, couscous, kamut, bulgur, durum, semolina, graham, triticale, einkorn, and all of their products contain gluten. Oats do not contain gluten, but they're often stored in the same facilities as gluten-containing grains, so if you buy oats, make sure that they are labeled gluten-free. Also note that avenin, a protein found in oats, can be problematic for some. Pay attention to your body, and if you suspect you have an issue with oats, eliminate them for the program. During reintroduction, you will know how your body responds. Brown rice, millet, amaranth, and quinoa are gluten-free grains.

The gluten molecule of today is different from what it was even a few generations ago. Selective breeding practices and modifications have yielded a molecule that is difficult for the body to break down, which ultimately results in an overstimulated immune system as well as dysfunction of the lining of the small intestine, creating an environment that is ripe for leaky gut. Gluten sensitivity remains one of the largest undiagnosed health problems in the United States today. Keep in mind that gluten is found in many shampoos, soaps, and other personal-care products as well. Read product labels carefully!

◎ **Dairy products.** All cow, goat, and sheep dairy products fall under the heading of *dairy products* and include milk, cheese, cream, half and half, and even fermented milk products such as yogurt, sour cream, and kefir. "Wait!" I can hear you exclaim, "I thought yogurt was great for digestive health!" Technically, it's the *bacteria* in yogurt that makes it good for you. However, sensitivity to the dairy protein casein, and lactose (dairy sugar), is rampant. In order to make sure this is not true for you, you will be using supplemental probiotics—in much higher doses than those found in yogurt—to support your gut flora while you are on the Gut Restoration Program.

◎ **Soy and soy products.** These have managed to worm their way into our food supply in a major way. Soy items are found in virtually all processed and packaged foods, and you can find soybean oil in many types of foods. In fact, Americans get most of their linoleic acid (a type of polyunsaturated fat) intake from soybean oil. For the duration of the Gut Restoration Program, you'll eliminate edamame, tofu, tempeh, soy milk, soy proteins, soy protein bars, soybean oil, soy sprinkles, and soy imitation meats from your diet. If you read labels carefully, you will notice that many products have lecithin in them that has been derived from soy. If you are in a pinch, it is okay to have lecithin from soy. Fermented soy, like tamari (wheat-free soy sauce) and miso, are the exceptions to this rule.

Soy is rough on the gastrointestinal system for a couple reasons. For one, soy contains protease inhibitors. Protease is the enzyme that breaks down proteins. As soy is ingested, protein digestion is inhibited. To add insult to injury, soy contains carbohydrates that are unrecognizable to the human digestive tract. This means that they are not broken down and digested. When large, unbroken proteins and carbohydrate molecules hit the small intestine, gas, bloating, and cramping are the result. Like other legumes, soy contains compounds called saponins and lectins that irritate the lining of the intestine.

◎ **Beans and legumes.** This group includes lentils and all varieties of beans and peanuts. I know many people love beans, particularly in Mexican food, but for anyone who has compromised GI function, it is disastrous to eat them. In addition to creating a lot of gas and bloating, beans and legumes contain lectins, phytates, and saponins, just like soy; and they worsen digestive function by irritating the lining of the small intestine, which in turn creates inflammation and impairs the absorption of nutrients.

◎ **Vegetables in the nightshade family (Solanaceae).** They contain a variety of compounds, but the ones we are interested in are a pair of alkaloids called solanine and chaconine. These two chemicals increase the permeability of the small intestine, triggering or inflaming leaky gut. The nightshades have also been implicated in the development of both osteo- and rheumatoid arthritis and can worsen symptoms of reflux. Tomatoes, white potatoes, bell pepper, cayenne pepper (note that black and white peppercorns are okay to eat), paprika, and eggplant are to be avoided for the duration of the program.

◎ **Refined white sugar and other sweeteners.** Products containing sugar, including baked goods, soda, and candy, are excluded during the program. In addition to having practically zero redeeming nutritional value, sugar aggravates the lining of the digestive tract, making the immune system more susceptible to viruses. It also feeds any pathogenic organisms you may have on board such as yeast, parasites, or troublesome bacteria. Sugar is addictive; and it can create mood swings, drain your energy, and worsen acne.

Before you get too excited about all the artificial sweeteners you think you'll be able to eat in place of sugar, while you're on the Gut Restoration Program, be aware that Splenda, Sweet'N Low, NutraSweet, and Equal can cause cravings, hunger, gas, and bloating and are also eliminated from the program. Even sugar alcohols such as maltitol should be avoided, as these cause gas and bloating. The natural sugar alcohol xylitol is well tolerated by some but not by everyone. You'll have to experiment and see what works best for you. Avoid honey, Karo syrup, agave nectar, barley malt, and rice syrup, as well.

Sweeteners that are OK to use during the program are stevia, in both powdered and liquid form, and coconut nectar and coconut (palm) sugar. Limit your intake of any of these sweeteners to one tablespoon or less per day. Note that people with yeast or dysbiosis issues are going to have to avoid coconut sugar and nectar as well.

◉ **Alcohol.** Beer, wine, hard spirits, and liquor are excluded altogether from the Gut Restoration Program. Alcohol is essentially metabolized as sugar, carrying with it empty calories that won't serve you well if you are trying to heal. Alcohol also slows the rate at which the cells that line the GI tract replace themselves and can exacerbate leaky gut. Don't worry, booze will be there for you at the end of four weeks.

Wolves in Sheeps' Clothing

In order to keep the program practical and as low stress as possible, the most common allergenic foods are targeted for removal. However, many people have sensitivities to an additional subset of foods. While these foods don't quite make the "big bullies" list, you should be aware of them and their potential to wreak digestive havoc.

If you begin the program and are not feeling better by the halfway point, consider elimination of one or more of these foods. Start by eliminating the "suspect" food you consume the most and see how you feel after a few days. If you are feeling better, you've found it. If not, try eliminating a different food.

◉ **Chia seeds.** Long touted as a digestive panacea for the gastrointestinal tract, they are anything but! In fact, chia seeds contain saponins and lectins, which can damage the lining of the intestine. Cut them out and watch your belly de-bloat.

- **Corn.** Like soy, it is found in virtually all processed food products. It can be particularly difficult for some people to digest. The vast majority of corn in the United States is GMO (genetically modified organism), and the safety studies are not there to back up its use.
- **Thickeners.** Carageenan, guar gum, xantham gum, and others can cause inflammation of the GI tract in some people. These products are often found in gluten-free baking mixes and products, and milk alternatives such as almond milk. Thickeners give products body and good mouth feel, but they can do a number on your gastrointestinal system.
- **Eggs.** The simple egg is problematic for some people. Although egg sensitivity is not as common as some other food sensitivities, it absolutely must be mentioned here.
- **Tree nuts.** Nuts, particularly almonds, are found in many foods and can be a source of woe for your belly. Most people with sensitivity to tree nuts will report that their mouth or eyes feel itchy after eating them, but this is not always the case.
- **Citrus fruit.** Lemons, oranges, limes, tangerines, grapefruit, clementines, etc. can be a hidden cause of digestive symptoms.
- **Strawberries.** These are another often-overlooked offender, particularly since many health-care providers recommend regular consumption of berries because of their many health benefits. However, medicine for one person can be poison for another.
- **Caffeine.** The ability to metabolize caffeine can vary by a thousand fold from one individual to the next. Some people can drink an entire pot of French-press coffee, top it off with a shot of espresso after dinner, and sleep like a baby that night, while others get heart palpitations and feel jumpy with just a little bit of caffeine in their system. Listen to your body. If you rely on caffeine for energy or if you aren't sure about how your body handles it, you may want to try removing it from your diet for the duration of the program (four weeks) to see how you feel.

Listen to What Your Body Is Telling You

How do you know if you're sensitive to a food that is not on one of the previous lists? The easiest answer is sometimes you just know. If you eat a food that consistently makes you feel unwell—even if it is tasty or supposed to be healthy—your body might not like it anyway. The important thing is to listen to what your body is telling you.

Testing for Food Allergies

Another way to find out if you are sensitive to particular foods is to be tested for food allergies. The results of testing can be confusing, however, because there are a couple ways to test allergic reactions that tell us different things. For example, someone may come into my clinic and proclaim that their doctor has tested him or her for food allergies, with the result that they "don't have any." I always ask: "Did you have your skin pricked or was blood drawn?" and 95 percent of the time they reply that their skin was pricked. It is important to understand that these testing methods are checks for two very different types of allergies.

The skin-prick test checks for a particular type of reaction that is driven by **IgE** (Immunoglobulin E) antibodies. Immunoglobulin E is known as the "evil" antibody because it creates acute, rapid onset, i.e., anaphylactic-type reactions like swelling of the eyes, face, lips, and throat, extreme congestion and runny nose, itchy, watery eyes, and difficulty breathing. These are the types of reactions that are going to drive you to look for some Benadryl and, in some cases, such as a peanut, shellfish, or bee allergy, necessitate that you carry an EpiPen. IgE allergies are one way you can have sensitivities to food but not the only way.

IgG antibodies drive a far more common—though less commonly tested—type of food sensitivity. IgG sensitivities are responsible for slowly accumulating, chronic, nebulous symptoms that can take up to 72 hours to manifest, unlike rapidly developing IgE reactions. Their effects are no less irksome, however, than their more dramatic and swift counterparts. It's a strong bet that almost everybody with a diagnosed digestive disorder or chronic gastrointestinal symptoms has a food sensitivity that they are not aware of.

IgG testing requires a blood draw, unlike the skin-prick test used to detect IgE antibodies. This type of test is available through your doctor or healthcare provider. If your doctor is unwilling to perform this test, you can order it online through Life Extension (see Resources, page 303) or shop around for a new doctor.

Testing for IgG sensitivities is not a requirement of the Gut Restoration Program. Most people will get results simply by avoiding the "big bullies" (see pages 73–77) in their diet. However, if you complete the program and still don't feel good, additional testing for food sensitivity—or something else, such as a hidden yeast or parasitic infection, may be warranted.

Eliminating Bacterial Imbalance and Infection

A prominent underlying theme in many chronic digestive symptoms and diagnosed disorders is the presence of subtle, insidious bacterial, yeast, or parasitic organisms that slowly create symptoms over time, unlike the immediate and dramatic symptoms of food poisoning or hemorrhagic *E. coli*. Contenders fall into several main categories: bacterial, yeast/fungal, and parasitic infection. Bacterial infection can be further teased out. It is possible to have harmful bacteria, such as *Helicobacter pylori*, *Enterobacter*, or *Clostridium difficile* on board. Or, you can be free of those nefarious characters and have a problem called dysbiosis, which occurs when there is an imbalance between good, beneficial bacteria and bad, potentially harmful bacteria. In dysbiosis, the scales are tipped in such a way that harmful bacteria or organisms are unable to be controlled by your normal flora and immune system and, thus, create symptoms. Chronic antibiotic use, diets low in protein and fiber and high in refined sugar, antacid use, and a history of using acid-blocking drugs predispose one to dysbiosis.

Bacterial Overgrowth in the Small Intestine

Sometimes, beneficial bacteria creep into areas where they don't belong. If they move upstream, set up shop in the small intestine, and start doing their job of fermenting, metabolizing, and multiplying, this is called small intestine bacterial overgrowth (SIBO)—a matter of having the right stuff in the wrong place (kind of like reflux!). SIBO can create symptoms of gas and bloating as well as intolerance to fiber, sugar, and probiotic supplements. Additionally, SIBO has been associated with long-term use of proton pump inhibitors and other acid-blocking drugs, restless legs syndrome, fibromyalgia, and IBS. All forms of dysbiosis are addressed on pages 217–218.

Yeast Overgrowth

Yeast overgrowth can manifest in a variety of ways that mimic food sensitivity and other gastrointestinal issues. The rub here is that small amounts of yeast are part of our normal flora. Problems arise when this population of yeast grows and remains unchecked. In this scenario, yeast overgrowth is a form of dysbiosis wearing another costume. In the case of unremitting symptoms that won't go away, in conjunction with a history of chronic urinary-tract infections (UTIs) or vaginal infections, alternating diarrhea and constipation, depression, sensitivities to multiple environmental agents, and worsening symptoms with the consumption of sugar, yeast overgrowth should be ruled out; if those symptoms are present, however, they should be addressed. Yeast eradication is specifically addressed in Chapter 17, "Candida" (see page 227).

Parasites

Most people associate parasitic infection with travel to exotic places or drinking dirty water, but the reality is that there are plenty of parasites here in the United States. Parasites are a hugely underestimated contributing factor and cause of gastrointestinal complaints. The standard method of detection for parasitic infection is an ova and parasite test, also called O and P. This test is sorely lacking in sensitivity and reach in its ability to detect parasites, however. In fact, the process, in which a small piece of stool is examined under a microscope as the clinician looks for something to float or swim by, is a bit like looking for a needle in a haystack: What if there aren't any parasites present in that particular bit of stool? What if you aren't shedding parasites at precisely that time? Consequently, O and P testing has a high rate of false negatives, which means you get the all-clear when in fact a parasite is present. Antigen or genetic testing is far more sensitive and accurate because it looks for genetic material in the stool that has been sloughed off by the parasite. The parasitic body does not have to be present in order for it to be detected by this test.

Cyclical symptoms that come in waves and wax and wane but never go away completely are key indicators of parasites. Night sweats and an unexplained high white-blood-cell count can be indicative of parasites. If your symptoms have developed or worsened after any type of travel, including camping, where you may have drunk water from a stream or other questionable source of clean water, you may have a parasitic infection. The protocol to extinguish parasites can be found in Chapter 15, "Dysbiosis" (see page 216).

Be mindful that many ordinary daily activities such as playing with pets or children in your garden or eating raw foods and salad greens that haven't been thoroughly washed can put you at risk for parasitic infection. This information is not meant to scare or gross you out but simply to make you more aware of the multiple avenues through which parasites can hitch a ride.

Testing for Parasitic Infection

If you are concerned that your body may be harboring a parasitic or a yeast or bacterial infection, you can confirm or rule out your suspicions with a comprehensive digestive stool analysis (CDSA). In addition to detecting pathogenic bacteria, yeast, and parasites, a CDSA will give you valuable information about the population of beneficial bacteria in your body and your digestive capacity, as well as indicate if there is any intestinal inflammation. CDSAs can be ordered through your doctor or your integrative health-care provider. The test costs about $350 and is sometimes covered by insurance.

Reducing Exposure to Gut-Harming Substances

It's a rough world out there—or at least it can be for our tender bellies. Around every corner, it seems, there are agents that are just waiting to exacerbate gut permeability, alter the balance of beneficial bacteria in the large intestine or alter the expression of our immune system and the balance of hormones, and otherwise create gastrointestinal signs and symptoms. It is just as important to remove or greatly minimize these components as it is to eliminate inflammatory foods and eradicate infection.

The Dangers of BPA

The first place to start cleaning up the environment around you is to eliminate exposure to a compound called bisphenol A. Also known as BPA, this compound is mostly found in plastics. Many of you are likely familiar with BPA and the splash it has been making in the media over these past few years. BPA is the new boogey monster in the world of public health. It grabs headlines for interrupting hormonal signaling and impairing brain development in newborn babies, but the damage it dishes out to the lining of the small intestine is just as problematic.

Luckily, BPA is getting easier and easier to avoid because enormous companies such as Gerber and Walmart are responding to consumer demand for BPA-free products by selling millions of plastic products, such as water bottles, pacifiers, and aluminum cans that are clearly labeled *BPA free.*

Reduce Your Exposure to Heavy Metals

Heavy metals such as mercury, lead, and aluminum can contribute to chronic gastrointestinal symptoms and blunt the ability of the small intestine to regenerate. Although they are not a commonly thought-of cause, heavy metals can also worsen heartburn and exacerbate all types of colitis, including inflammatory bowel disease.

We are exposed to metals in the air we breathe, in food and water, and in mercury from tooth fillings. Strategies to reduce heavy-metal exposure can start with minimizing the use of canned foods. You may also want to consider installing a water filtration system under your kitchen sink, or even a whole house filtration system, which can cost less than $500 to install and about $100 per year in filters. Of course, in a pinch, you can simply get a water pitcher that has a good filter, such as a Brita.

Another easy trick to reduce your exposure to heavy metals is to put an air filter in your bedroom, work area, or wherever you spend the majority of your day—or move it around with you. Soil is contaminated with metals from car exhaust that settles into the ground. As you walk on these contaminated surfaces, the compounds get on your shoes and are then tracked into the house. In order to avoid this contamination, it helps to remove your shoes before entering the house. If you are not ventilating your home daily and do not use air filters, heavy metals from exhaust can get into the air your breathe. Indoor air quality is notoriously worse than outdoor air quality, largely due to the presence of a high concentration of metals. Air filters can cost anywhere from $40 to thousands of dollars, depending on size and quality. Even a small air filter, however, can help reduce the amount of metals you breathe in.

Cosmetics, Cleaning, and Personal-Care Products

Cosmetics, particularly liquid foundation, mascara, and lipstick, contain heavy metals and other compounds that can be problematic for sensitive individuals. If you use cosmetics regularly, you my want to consider switching to mineral-based products, such as Mineral Fusion, ZuZu, and DeVita, which are available now, thanks to consumers who requested them.

You may also want to consider switching to natural cleaning and personal-care products. Dish soap, laundry detergent, body wash, toothpaste, hand soap, shampoo, and a host of other products contain the surfactants sodium lauryl sulfate (SLS) and dextran sulfate sodium (DSS). These compounds are used to induce colitis in lab rats—to enable researchers to look for cures for IBD, ironically—and are well-documented irritants of the GI system. There are several options out there for non-SLS and non-DSS–based personal-care and home products. It is as simple as reading labels.

Dryer sheets are highly irritating. They contain a slew of compounds that are bothersome to the central nervous system and upper respiratory system and are capable of inducing headaches, nausea, and stomach cramps. Instead, opt for products from companies such as Seventh Generation, Method, If You Care, and the 365 brand from Whole Foods.

Opioids and Antibiotics

Finally, a couple of classes of drugs are worth bringing to your attention because of the enormous impact they have on gastrointestinal health. (These are covered in more detail in Chapter 6, "Medications and Digestive Health," page 52.) Opioids, including painkillers such as codeine, fentanyl, Vicodin, Percocet, oxycodone, and morphine have significant effects on the digestive system. These drugs remove pain but leave debilitating constipation in their wake.

Unless they are absolutely necessary and no other options exist and you are under strict doctor's orders to continue with them, consider seeking alternatives to opiates. Listen to your body and your doctor first.

Another class of drugs that interferes with gastrointestinal function is antibiotics. Antibiotics are highly effective at killing bacteria, and that is a good thing. However, they are nondiscriminatory, so they kill the beneficial bacteria that are centrally important for tip-top gastrointestinal and immune health, as well.

If you are taking antibiotics, it may be best to wait until you have completed your course before starting the Gut Restoration Program. If that is not feasible, double your dose of probiotics for a length of time that lasts three times as long as your antibiotic course (for example, if you're on a one-week antibiotic course, take probiotics for three weeks, starting the same week as the antibiotic course). You can, and should, take probiotics and antibiotics together. Taking the two simultaneously will help reduce the side effects of antibiotics, such as diarrhea, cramping, and pain, without reducing the efficacy of the antibiotic.

Step 2. Take a Probiotic

We humans have a symbiotic relationship with the bacteria, all 100 trillion of them, that live in our large intestine. This mutually beneficial relationship has developed over the millennia and serves both parties well. Intestinal bacteria provide innumerable services for us, ranging from digestive and immune to metabolic functions.

Sometimes, our bacteria need a little outside help to boost morale and keep all systems running efficiently. That is when supplemental probiotics come in. Probiotics can help prop up and fill in the gaps in our microbiota, even if they don't stick around forever.

Probiotics 101

All probiotics are not created equal. When selecting a probiotic, there are several key elements to keep in mind:

- For adults, look for a product that primarily has *Lactobacillus* and *Bifidobacteria* strains. Some product manufacturers get very fancy and pack in multiple strains, and that is fine, but make sure *Lactobacillus* and *Bifidobacteria* are prominently featured.
- For babies and toddlers, look for a product that includes *B. infantis*, as well as *Lactobacillus* and other *Bifidobacteria* strains.
- Because probiotics can be a hidden source of allergens, look for products that have not been grown in soy or dairy mediums. The label should say *hypoallergenic*. Using a probiotic that contains dairy or soy ingredients defeats the purpose of avoiding allergenic foods, so make sure you read those labels!
- For the duration of the program, take 100 billion CFUs daily with breakfast. This dose of probiotics is going to be higher than you may be accustomed to taking, because of its therapeutic use in the program. If this dose makes you feel gassy, bloated, or otherwise uncomfortable, start with 20 billion CFUs

and double the dose every other day until you are up to 100 billion CFUs. If you are unable to reach that level because of discomfort, there is a good chance that you have SIBO, or some form of dysbiosis, and you should initiate the protocol found in Chapter 15, "Dysbiosis" (see page 216).

What about Prebiotics?

Beneficial bacteria have to eat too, right? Prebiotics are a group of food compounds and soluble fibers that are used to feed the beneficial flora in your large intestine.

Inulin, fructooligosaccharide (FOS), arabinogalactan, and fructans are fancy names for prebiotic fibers. Prebiotics help the beneficial bacteria with their chores of fermentation and digestion of food, increasing the absorption of nutrients. They increase the local production of short-chain fatty acids (SCFA), a major fuel source for enterocytes, the cells that line the gastrointestinal tract. By ensuring that beneficial bacteria are well fed and producing energy, prebiotics indirectly promote optimal regeneration, differentiation, and integrity of the cells that line the gut wall. This is very good news for anyone who has any type of digestive problem. To top it all off, prebiotic fibers have been shown to decrease the risk for colon cancer.

There is some debate in complementary and integrative circles about whether probiotic supplements should also contain prebiotics. There's a short answer to that debate: no, they shouldn't. The addition of prebiotics to probiotic formulations can create a lot of gas and bloating, creating confusion for people who are trying to get to the root of their digestive issues. If you eat vegetables and fruit every day, you are consuming sufficient quantities of prebiotics to feed your hungry bacteria. Bottom line: Eat your prebiotics—don't use them as supplements.

Foods that are particularly rich in prebiotics include artichokes, Jerusalem artichokes/sunchokes, jicama, chicory, dandelion greens, oats and oat bran, garlic, leeks and onions, green tea, asparagus, and bananas. Incorporating these foods into your diet will provide a steady stream of prebiotic fuel to keep your gut flora happy.

Step 3. Boost Digestive Ability

Enzymes, acid, and bile facilitate the breakdown of proteins, starches, and fats into small compounds. These small compounds are then easily absorbed into the blood, don't irritate the small intestine, and don't provoke an unfavorable immune response. Digestive capacity is central to a healthy gastrointestinal system. You could be eating the most perfect, appropriate diet for your body, but if you lack the ability to break it down, all of that perfect food won't be absorbed and your body won't be functioning at its best.

All About Enzymes

Digestive enzymes are primarily produced by the pancreas and found in small amounts in saliva and the small intestine. Digestive enzymes break down proteins, fats, and carbohydrates into their constituent amino acids, fatty acids, and sugars.

Enzymes are an integral part of the digestive capacity of the body. Without enzymes, your body's ability to break down and absorb proteins, carbohydrates, fats, and other nutrients is compromised. Eating processed foods and eating foods that you are sensitive to, along with chronic stress, lack of sleep, and aging are all causes of lowered enzyme production by the body. Supplementing with digestive enzymes ensures that your body will have enough enzymes to break up macronutrients and, thus, absorb nutrition from the food you eat.

Finding the Right Enzymes

Luckily, enzymes have a long shelf life and retain their stability for roughly three years, so you don't have to worry as much about their longevity as you would about probiotics, which have a shorter shelf life. Nevertheless, a trip down the "digestive health" aisle at any health food store can be confusing because there are so many enzyme products out there. Here's what to look for:

- **A plant-based enzyme formula that is clearly labeled as such.** Enzymes are small protein molecules that split up larger macronutrients into their constituent parts for easy absorption and assimilation. Supplemental enzymes are derived from either plant, fungal, or animal (typically bovine) sources. This is an important consideration for vegans.
- **An enzyme blend rather than single enzymes.** In order to best mimic the enzymatic output of the pancreas, supplement your diet with a broad range of

enzymes. There are many blends that have multiple enzymes rolled into one
product.

- **Enzymes that list activity levels, instead of milligrams.** On the labels,
  you will notice that most products have units such as USP, IAU, DU,
  HUT, and so on in place of milligrams or micrograms. These units signify
  an activity level of the enzyme rather than a quantifiable unit. If you buy
  a product that lists milligrams, there is no way of knowing if there are any
  active enzymes in it at all. All rules have their exceptions, however. Some
  enzymes products that are available only through health-care providers
  quantify their enzymes in milligrams, and are tested for enzymatic activity.
  If in doubt, stick to activity levels. At a minimum, choose a product that
  contains at least these enzymes:
    - **Protease—10,000 USP (protein digestion)**
    - **Amylase—10,000 USP (carbohydrate digestion)**
    - **Lipase—2,000 USP (fat digestion)**
- **A product that includes an assortment of other enzymes.** It should be
  mixed with protease, amylase, and lipase enzymes, including peptidase,
  galactosidase (this is the enzyme that's in Beano—a product that is a far cry
  from a comprehensive digestive enzyme formula), invertase, glucoamylase,
  diastase, lactase, glucoamylase, phytase, cellulase, beta-glucanase, and pepsin.
  For the duration of the Gut Restoration Program, take two capsules of digestive enzymes with meals. They are typically small, easy to swallow, and very well
  tolerated.

Stomach-Acid Basics

Hydrochloric acid (HCl) is secreted by the stomach and breaks down protein molecules. It acts as a defense against pathogenic organisms such as bacteria, yeast,
and viruses. HCl is required to absorb calcium, iron, vitamin C, vitamin B12, and
beta-carotene. HCl plays a role in the absorption of magnesium, zinc, chromium,
copper, vanadium, selenium, and manganese.

An immense energetic effort is required on the part of the stomach cells to
produce adequate stomach acid. With age, stress, poor nutrition, and digestive
complaints such as leaky gut, making enough acid becomes difficult, and digestive
power suffers.

Do I Need to Take Supplemental Acid?

One of the major aspects of digestive capacity is adequate stomach-acid production. Acid is important for the breakdown of proteins and other macronutrients, and for absorption of vitamins and other micronutrients needed to maintain proper pH balance of the digestive system and reduce the likelihood of infection.

For most people, a four-week course of supplemental acid is well tolerated. There are a couple of notable exceptions: if you have an active ulcer or gastritis, supplemental acid is contraindicated. If you have a history of ulcer or gastritis and are unsure if you have healed, do not take supplemental acid.

You could greatly benefit from taking supplemental acid if these are some of your symptoms: frequent belching and bloating, particularly following meals; a feeling of fullness for an extended time after meals, or getting full quickly; low appetite; nausea in the morning, or after taking supplements; weak and brittle nails that chip easily; undigested food in the stool; a history of iron deficiency or vitamin B deficiency; anemia; a history of taking acid-blocking drugs.

How to Take Supplemental Acid

Supplemental acid is available either singly or in combination with digestive enzymes. If you are confident that you are going to take supplemental acid, it is probably easier to get a product that contains both acid and enzymes. Most commonly, betaine HCl is the form of acid found in most products.

Start out with 200 milligrams–500 milligrams of betaine HCl with major meals. If, upon taking it, you experience warmth or flushing in the stomach or over your skin, heart palpitations, or burning in the esophagus or stomach, please discontinue using betaine HCl. These symptoms indicate that you are producing sufficient stomach acid and do not need to supplement it any further.

Supplemental acid helps stimulate the stomach to fire up its own production of acid. In this scenario, you may notice that it gives you the listed symptoms after taking betaine HCl for a couple of weeks. This is your body's way of letting you know it has awakened—it is doing its job and supplementation is no longer necessary.

If a week or more has gone by without feeling warmth or any other symptoms, and you are still experiencing bloating, gas, or other low-acid symptoms, increase the dose of betaine HCl to 500–1,000 milligrams, and take it with major meals for the remainder of the program. If you experience symptoms of warmth, flushing, or palpitations, discontinue supplemental acid.

Bile Basics

Bile is produced by the liver and stored in the gallbladder until a fat-containing meal is eaten. The gallbladder then squeezes and propels bile into the stomach, where it does its job. Bile acts very much like soap, breaking apart and dispersing fat into smaller and smaller molecules in a process called emulsification. Emulsification makes it easy for fat-digesting enzymes to go to work. When gallbladder function is impaired, fats become difficult to digest and can trigger uncomfortable symptoms like pain and nausea.

The body uses bile to eliminate toxins and metabolic by-products that are not readily dissolved in water. When something is easily dissolved in water, it gets into the blood and is filtered by the liver. Compounds that don't dissolve well in water are handled in part by bile. Bile "packages" these compounds and sends them to the intestine to be pooped out.

For people who no longer have a gallbladder, supplementation with 200–400 milligrams of bile at mealtimes is recommended. Many enzyme products contain bile. While there are vegetarian formulas for supplemental bile, many of them are derived from ox bile.

Step 4. Repair the Gut Lining

Reparation of the lining of the gastrointestinal wall is the icing on the cake in the Gut Restoration Program. If this step is neglected, no matter how perfect your diet, the addition of probiotics and digestive aids is going to fall short. A door will be left open for infection, inflammation, and immune dysfunction, along with the potential for food sensitivities and the never-ending perpetuation of symptoms.

The lining of the small intestine plays a particularly important role in digestive health. The small intestine is where the vast majority of nutrients are absorbed. When it is injured or compromised a smoldering, chronic immune response is initiated, eventually creating leaky gut and impairing absorption of nutrients. The cells that line the small intestine have very rapid turnover, but if the inflammatory fire is not snuffed out, turnover time can lengthen, leaving more holes in the system. Leaky gut is self-perpetuating until the right ingredients for healing are introduced.

The major objective for repairing the digestive tract is to decrease the permeability or "leakiness" of the small intestine. This in turn will quell abnormal immune response to food and blunt the release of inflammatory compounds locally and body-wide. Through the reduction of inflammation, pain, irritation, and other symptoms are reduced. Immune function begins to normalize and self-regulate. It is possible that autoimmune responses will begin to abate. The lining of the gastrointestinal tract will be soothed. With the restoration of structure, appropriate function will follow, and you will feel better.

Gut-Healing Nutrients and How to Take Them

There are many good options for gastrointestinal repair. Look for a product that contains all or most of the compounds you need. The best formulas are going to combine amino acids, vitamins, minerals, herbs, and other compounds. Some of the best products on the market are GI Restore by Metabolic Effect, GI Revive by Designs for Health, and Intestinal Complex by Pharmax. Here is a list of the major players that restore the integrity of the gut wall:

- **L-glutamine** is the preferred fuel for the cells that line the gut wall. These cells seek out glutamine when food comes through the intestines. Glutamine is the base for reparation of the gastrointestinal tract.

- **Glutamine** is anti-catabolic. In other words, it prevents cells from breaking down prematurely, thereby helping cellular growth, differentiation, and regeneration. Glutamine decreases leaky gut by repairing the tight junctions of cells that line the small intestine. Remember that tight junctions are the structures that button cells together, ensuring the integrity of the gut wall.

  Dose: 4,000–8,000 milligrams daily, in divided doses (2,000–4,000 milligrams twice daily)

- **Zinc carnosine** protects the lining of the gastrointestinal tract, decreases inflammation, and protects against ulceration of the stomach and intestines. It is important for the optimal production of hydrochloric acid in the stomach, which protects against *H. pylori* and other types of infection, and is a cornerstone for protein breakdown. Zinc carnosine buffers the negative effects of anti-inflammatory drugs on the gastrointestinal system.

  Dose: 75–100 milligrams daily, in divided doses (50 milligrams twice daily)

- **Methylsulfonylmethane (MSM)** quells inflammation and reduces the release of histamine. It assists in building collagen and helps reconstruct the gastrointestinal lining. As an added bonus, parasites detest this sulfur-rich compound.

Dose: 100 milligrams daily, in divided doses (50 milligrams twice daily)

◎ **Quercetin** is a bioflavonoid and powerful anti-inflammatory agent. It is particularly effective against long-standing inflammation. It stabilizes cells that release histamine and other irritating components, making it particularly useful for those who suffer from seasonal allergies. Quercetin acts as an antioxidant, reducing damage to the lining of the intestinal wall.

Dose: 100 milligrams daily, in divided doses (50 milligrams twice daily)

◎ **N-acetyl glucosamine (NAG)** is a building block for the soft tissue of the intestinal wall. It acts like mortar that is slathered between the bricks of your digestive system to build a healthy, strong intestinal lining. NAG will directly improve leaky gut.

Budding research shows that NAG also helps calm autoimmune response, making it particularly appropriate for those with autoimmune conditions. **Note:** Many sources of NAG are derived from shellfish and would not be appropriate for anyone with a shellfish allergy. Practice due diligence and read labels.

Dose: 1,000–1,200 milligrams daily, in divided doses (500–600 milligrams twice daily)

◎ **Herbs.** There are several herbal options for gastrointestinal repair. These herbs help relax and soothe irritated tissue, coat the lining of the intestine, reduce gas and bloating, and decrease ulceration and inflammation. There are multiple formulas, such as GI Restore by Metabolic Effect and GI Revive by Designs for Health, that contain many or all of the herbs in the following list. Make sure that the formula you use includes as many of these herbs as possible:

  ◎ **Deglycyrrhizinated licorice (DGL).** It has one of the longest histories of use in gastrointestinal complaints. It helps to coat and soothe the digestive tract. DGL helps form a protective barrier against inflammation and contains antioxidant properties.

  Dose: 400 milligrams daily, in divided doses (200 milligrams twice daily)

  ◎ **Aloe Vera.** This plant has an extensive history and use in healing the digestive system. It acts as a balm to inflamed tissues, helps with regularity, and acts as a food source to friendly bacteria. Aloe suppresses the growth of yeast and harmful bacteria. It makes the immune system more responsive to pathogens and decreases autoimmune action.

Dose: 300 milligrams daily, in divided doses (150 milligrams twice daily)

◎ **Slippery elm bark.** Slippery elm belongs to the mucilaginous ("slippery") class of herbs. Slippery elm and other mucilaginous herbs cover the wall of the digestive tract with a protective barrier. This barrier not only protects the system from irritants but also nourishes, reduces inflammation, and heals wounds. As an added bonus, slippery elm tastes pretty good too.

Dose: 200 milligrams daily, in divided doses (100 milligrams twice daily)

◎ **Chamomile.** This pretty little flower is best known as a soothing before-bed tea, and it has major implications in gastrointestinal repair. Chamomile reduces spasm and cramping. It dissolves and removes gas from the system, and reduces bloating and gas pains.

Dose: 100 milligrams daily, in divided doses (50 milligrams twice daily)

◎ **Marshmallow, cat's claw, and okra.** Like Slippery elm, these herbs have mucilaginous qualities. They act as an emollient on the intestinal wall, creating a protective barrier. The barrier allows for healing of ulcerated or inflamed tissues and reduces sensitivity to gastric juices and inflammatory compounds. These herbs decrease spasms and improve digestive comfort.

Dose: 100 milligrams daily of each, in divided doses (50 milligrams twice daily)

◎ **Mucin.** Your gut secretes this protein. Harmful bacteria, other invaders, and toxins are neutralized in part by mucin. Its non-inflammatory immune action does not create swelling, heat, redness, or pain. Mucin coats the lining of the intestine to create a protective barrier.

Dose: 200 milligrams daily, in divided doses (100 milligrams twice daily)

◎ **Citrus pectin and prune powder.** These gentle, non-caustic fibers aid in regularity of bowel movements without being habit forming. Beneficial bacteria feed on both citrus pectin and prune powder, and the powders are safe for long-term use. Citrus pectin aids in cell division and regeneration, making it helpful for healing leaky gut. You may choose either or use both.

Citrus Pectin Dose: 1,000 milligrams per day, in divided doses (500 milligrams twice daily)

Prune Powder Dose: 100–200 milligrams per day, in divided doses (50–100 milligrams twice daily)

Step 5. Lifestyle Changes

Learning ways to de-stress and soothe your digestive system is crucial for restoring optimal digestive function. Stress creates imbalance in the nervous system, disrupts the ability to have regular bowel movements, and intensifies pain and other symptoms.

Bringing Harmony to Your Second Brain

The gastrointestinal system has a mind of its own. It is densely studded with nerve cells that help with the operation of digestion. Collectively, this set of cells is known as the enteric nervous system (ENS). The ENS is referred to as the second brain because it is capable of functioning independently of the brain while carrying out the task of digestion. A major responsibility of the ENS is the regulation of peristalsis, the rhythmic muscular contraction that propels food down the gastrointestinal tract toward its final destination—the toilet. When peristalsis is disordered, constipation, diarrhea, or a mix of these ensues.

Multiple factors can disrupt the ENS and peristalsis, including stress, food sensitivities, allergenic foods, dysbiosis, low beneficial flora, infection, and environmental agents.

Many of these elements are addressed within the Gut Restoration Program. One of the best behavioral interventions for the regulation of bowel function is to create a bathroom routine. At the same time each day, take several minutes to sit quietly on the toilet during the time you would like to have a bowel movement. Don't strain or force, simply sit. Over time, this routine trains the body to "go."

Balancing the Sympathetic and Parasympathetic Branches of the Nervous System

In Chapter 3, "The Digestive Players," the sympathetic and parasympathetic branches of the nervous system were explained (see page 15). The sympathetic branch is responsible for "fight or flight" reactions and is activated under stress. Its counterpart is the parasympathetic branch, which helps us relax, rest, and digest. Balancing the two branches of our nervous system is crucial for optimal gastrointestinal function.

In times of unremitting stress and long-term pain or digestive disturbance, the sympathetic branch becomes dominant, greatly suppressing optimal digestion. Under these circumstances, it is important to increase the function of the parasympathetic nervous system.

There are several options to consider while bringing the two branches of the nervous system back into balance. Perhaps the single most important factor is sleep. Getting enough sleep acts like a reset button for stress hormones and activates the parasympathetic nervous system.

Tips for Great Sleep

- Maintain a regular sleep-wake cycle. Try to go to bed and get up at roughly the same time each day. A deviation of an hour or two on the weekend is OK.
- Be in bed before 11:00 p.m., if possible. Research suggests that going to bed before this time promotes the best hormonal environment for sleep, regeneration, and even fat burning.
- Turn off all electronics at least 30 minutes before bed. The light from laptops, smartphones, and television is stimulating to the brain and releases compounds to keep you awake.
- Create a sleeping environment that promotes deep, restful slumber. The bedroom should be cool and dark. Invest in some light-blocking shades if necessary. Clear clutter such as stacks of paper and other piles of "stuff" from the bedroom. Consider a fan, white-noise machine, or app if you are a light sleeper. White noise helps drown out background noise.
- Have a bedtime routine. This could include taking a warm shower, reading an enjoyable book, or meditating.

Other Options for Getting a Great Night's Sleep

- Yoga, Tai Chi, and meditation are good tools to activate parasympathetic nervous system function.
- A thirty- to sixty-minute morning walk acts as a meditation if you take the time to enjoy the sights, sounds, textures, and smells of the outside world. A leisurely morning walk also helps to balance cortisol, a major stress hormone.
- It is also possible to supplement your diet with herbs and nutrients that boost the production of the neurotransmitter gamma-aminobutyric acid (GABA), a major whole-body, feel-good neurotransmitter that is boosted by 100–400 milligrams of 4-amino-3-phenylbutyric acid before bed. Herbs such as skullcap, valerian root, passionflower, and kava kava promote GABA release and function. These herbs are found singly or in blends as tinctures,

in capsules, or in tea. It is best to experiment with these herbs one by one to see how your body responds to them. Tinctures tend to be stronger than tea. Until you've assessed your response to these herbs, which can have sedative qualities, take them at night when you don't have to be productive.

Progressive Relaxation Technique

Try this simple technique for relaxing your entire body any time of day or just before sleep. Find a comfortable position. Either sitting in a well-supported position or lying on your back works well. Spend a few moments noticing and deepening your breath. Beginning with the top of your head, focus your attention on one part of your body at a time, consciously releasing any "holding" or tension in that one area, i.e., release and relax your scalp, then your face, then your throat, etc., taking as much time as you need with each part of our body until you have moved all the way down to the soles of your feet. It can help to imagine that these body parts are heavy and warm, sinking or melting into the chair, bed, or wherever you're resting. If you wish, you can contract the muscles in each area of your body for one or two seconds first, before letting go into relaxation. This is particularly helpful if you aren't sure what it feels like when a body part is physically relaxed. When you have completed the whole progression, continue resting quietly for a few minutes before transitioning to the rest of the day or evening.

CHAPTER 9

The Meal Plan
and Recipes

The only thing you really have to do for the healing gut-restoration meal plan is to avoid high-risk foods and incorporate some of the suggested support foods for four weeks. That's all. Because some of the foods on the elimination list are staples for many people, we have created a sample meal plan, including forty-five tasty, easy recipes, to give you an idea of how manageable this month can be without those staples. While there is nothing magical about this particular menu, it conforms perfectly to the Gut Restoration Program guidelines and may make it easier for you to follow them. It is also designed to give you a great balance of macronutrients (carbohydrates, fats, and proteins) and keep your blood sugar nice and stable which, in addition to all the health and digestion benefits that confers, will also help keep cravings for unnecessary sugars in check.

Avoid These Foods
- All nightshades, including white potatoes (sweet potatoes are fine), tomatoes, sweet and hot peppers, eggplant, tomatillos, tamarinos, pepinos, pimentos, paprika, and cayenne peppers
- Dairy, including butter
- Gluten, including wheat, spelt, rye, barley, and oats (unless certified gluten-free)
- Soy, including soy protein, tofu, soy protein isolates (in snack foods), and soy sauce (small amounts of fermented soy, as in rice miso or gluten-free tamari sauce, are permitted)
- Legumes, including all beans, and peanuts
- All sugars except stevia, erythritol (Truvia) and small amounts of palm sugar, or coconut nectar

Include These Foods

- Artichokes/sunchokes. Canned artichokes should be in olive oil, not soy; artichoke hearts should be packed in canola oil.
- Bone broth, including chicken, beef, fish, etc.
- Cabbage. Salads, soups, steamed cabbage, cabbage rolls, and sauerkraut are all suitable preparations.
- Coconut, including fresh coconut, coconut water, unsweetened chipped coconut, unsweetened shredded coconut, coconut milk, coconut butter, and coconut oil
- Fermented foods, including sauerkraut, fermented pickles, coconut yogurt, coconut kefir, etc.
- Okra (any preparation)
- Onions/garlic (any preparation)
- Protein (non-soy and non-bean), including non-soy vegan protein powder, meat, poultry, seafood, eggs, etc., preferably pasture raised
- Pumpkin (Any preparation is fine.)
- Turmeric/curcumin

Adding Superfoods to the Gut Restoration Menu

By choosing gut-friendly foods that pack a healthy punch, it is possible to speed up your healing process. Foods that specifically nourish and support the gastrointestinal system are easier than you think to incorporate into your daily or weekly diet.

The gastrointestinal all-stars detailed in the following pages have met several criteria. They provide energy while soothing and protecting the gastrointestinal system. These foods nourish the beneficial bacteria residing in the large intestine and keep pathogens at bay. Many are a source of gentle fiber, thus improving regularity. These gastrointestinal superfoods reduce local irritation and inflammation.

It is important to listen to your body first. If there is a food on the list that you know you don't tolerate well, skip it.

Coconut and coconut products. These produces include fresh coconut, coconut water, unsweetened chipped coconut, unsweetened shredded coconut, coconut milk, coconut butter, and coconut oil. Coconut is rich in short-chain fatty acids (SCFA). SCFAs are readily used as an immediate source of energy by the cells that line the GI tract. There is a surprisingly dense amount of fiber in coconut (a table-spoon of shredded coconut contains almost a gram of fiber). Coconut products also include the antiviral, antimicrobial compounds lauric acid and monolaurin, which protect the body from a wide variety of infections.

Leeks and onions. These foods are high in the anti-inflammatory bioflavo-noid quercetin. Onions are one of the most jam-packed food sources of quercetin available. Leeks and onions also have a slippery quality that is characteristic of gut-friendly foods. This slipperiness helps to coat the intestines, soothing inflamed tissues and protecting against further irritation.

Sweet potato and pumpkin. These orange foods are chock-full of beta-carotene, the precursor to vitamin A. Vitamin A promotes optimal cell regenera-tion and immune function, lending itself well to gut restoration. Pumpkin and sweet potato are great sources of gentle fiber and are low glycemic-index carbohy-drates. They won't spike your blood sugar.

Cabbage. The humble cabbage is fabulous for the gastrointestinal system because it is rich in glutamine. It contains sulfur-containing compounds that are protective against cancer. Cabbage has abundant phytonutrients—plant chemicals that have a broad range of positive health benefits—including antioxidants. Taking cabbage juice for ulcers and other gastrointestinal complaints is a long-standing folk remedy. Take it to heart and reap the many health benefits of eating cabbage!

Fermented foods. With the exclusion of dairy products from the gut-restoration menu, there is still a good selection of fermented foods to eat and enjoy. Fermented foods, often used in small amounts as condiments, supply the body with probiotics and enzymes and can improve the digestibility of a meal. Fermented foods protect the integrity of the small intestine, aid in the absorp-tion of vitamins and minerals, and are inherently antimicrobial. Sauerkraut (cab-bage); traditionally fermented pickled vegetables (pickles, olives, and capers); umeboshi plums; Thai fish sauce; amazake (rice drink); and fermented coconut products are examples of foods to be incorporated into the diet. A word to the wise, however: if you have a yeast infection or sensitivity to histamine, your condition may be aggravated by these foods, and you should minimize their use—always listen to your body!

Artichokes. Regular artichokes and Jerusalem artichokes (also known as sunchokes) are fiber superstars. All artichokes have ample amounts of prebiotic fiber, an essential food for your beneficial bacteria. Artichokes also contain soluble and insoluble fiber, which gently aid bowel regularity.

Okra. Common in the South, it may not be eaten quite as much in other parts of the country. If you open an okra pod, you'll discover its stringy and slippery insides. Okra is high in mucilaginous compounds that are capable of soothing the GI tract and reducing inflammation.

Protein. All biological systems are built with this structural framework, and the GI system is no different. Protein ensures that your gut lining will be appropriately constructed and that there will be enough building materials for enzymes. Adequate protein intake is crucial for immune function. Compounds that are used by the immune cells to communicate with each other and immunoglobulin (antibodies) are made from protein. If protein is lacking, our bodies turn to a stored source—muscle tissue—and break it down, making it difficult for our bodies to heal and function in an optimal way.

Bone Broth. Rich in vitamins, minerals, and the building blocks of collagen, bone broth builds up soft tissues. It is extremely nutritive and great for people with colitis, inflammatory bowel disease, and diverticulitis—especially in the middle of a flare. It is gentle and easy to absorb and assimilate.

Turmeric/Curcumin. This brilliant orange spice disrupts inflammation and helps soothe the GI tract. If you have inflammatory bowel disease, colitis, or colorectal cancer, be sure to add both curcumin and turmeric to your diet. Curcumin is a constituent of turmeric and is more readily absorbed into the bloodstream. Turmeric stays in the intestine, coating it like a soothing paint, and reducing inflammation. It's a one-two punch against inflammation. Curcumin aids in antioxidant production in addition to being a potent antioxidant in itself.

Prunes. The wisdom of our grandparents is well founded. Prunes are a fabulous source of very gentle, nonirritating, constipation-relieving fiber. Prunes are also a rich source of antioxidants, which helps reduce local inflammation in the gut. As a side note, prunes are also fabulous for bone health.

More Information about the Menus

All of the evening meals on the gut-restoration menu serve four, unless there are "built-in" leftovers for another meal or two. Making extra servings of certain entrées is a great strategy for reducing your time in the kitchen. With the exception of the special Sunday breakfast recipe for Egg and Portobello Florentine (see page 122), all breakfast and lunch suggestions are single servings.

Batching

If you aren't feeding a family, divide dinner recipes in half, when applicable, and freeze any entrée leftovers that aren't called for in the meal plan later in the week. Well-frozen leftovers will last for up to three months and can be used as supplemental meals, even after you complete the program. To freeze prepared meals, follow these steps:

- Store leftovers in the refrigerator overnight in freezer-safe containers (preferably tempered glass, such as Pyrex) with rubber lids.
- In the morning, remove any condensation from inside the lid and snugly cover the entire surface of the food with freezer-safe plastic wrap (to minimize air contact), then snap the lid over the plastic. This will help minimize the formation of ice crystals and prevent freezer burn.
- Place the prepared food in an open area in the freezer. You want the food to freeze as quickly as possible to ensure the formation of the smallest possible ice crystals. Once the food is frozen solid, you can stack it among other freezer items.
- To defrost the food, remove it from the freezer after dinner the night before you wish to eat it and let it thaw for 24 hours in the fridge. Microwave thawing is uneven, and thawing food on the countertop is dangerous (it can allow bacterial pathogens to multiply rapidly).
- The next night, heat the leftovers the way you would heat any other food.
- **A final note:** Salad vegetables do not freeze well because their water content is so high; they turn to mush when thawed. Only freeze entrées that are made primarily from meats, poultry, seafood, and hardy veggies.

The Gut Restoration Program is not about either calorie restriction or overindulgence. Everyone's portion needs are unique. A large, fit man in his twenties will need more calories than a small, sedentary woman in her sixties, so make adjustments to the program's meal and snack portions to suit your particular metabolic needs. Again, there is nothing rigid about the meal plan—customize it to fit your lifestyle. To further support your digestive healing process, the menu is relatively low in grains (including corn), nuts, and seeds. You may also notice that there are no flour-based foods.

You will find that the recipes are all quite easy, varied, and tasty, and most of them are quick to prepare, as well. You may experience a period of adjustment as your taste buds get accustomed to ingredient substitutions and the lack of some familiar ingredients, such as heavy sugars. However, the shift will happen rapidly and there are several comforting options on the menu to replace favorites such as pizza and ice cream.

Setting Yourself Up for Success

Whether you decide to use the gut-restoration menu plan or create your own, you will need to set aside some time on the weekend to prepare what you are going to eat each week. On Saturday, spend a little time looking over the week's menu. Make a list of any ingredient substitutions you may want to make, add seasonal fruit to your list, if you like, and then do your shopping on Saturday or Sunday for the following week.

Before you start the week, look over the recipes and make a note of anything that will require advance prep, such as cold tea, frozen bananas, marinades, or setting up a slow cooker on a particular day. Sunday is a great time to do a little preparatory kitchen work. You can make a big salad base and/or dressing for the week, a batch of tasty snacks to nosh on throughout the week, or a big pot of homemade Bone Broth (see recipe on page 160).

Support Tips for Digestive Health

If you are like the average American, you are probably not spending a lot of time in the kitchen. Eating for digestive health may mean more cooking than you're used to. The gut-restoration meal plan is set up to reduce the actual amount of time you spend cooking by providing recipes that can be doubled and ingredients that can be used in one, two, or even three additional meals or snacks. However, you need to prepare yourself for a lifestyle change. As you may have discovered from years and maybe decades of eating foods that don't work well for you, convenience foods are generally not good for your gut.

◎ **Variety.** If you are used to eating the same foods over and over, this meal plan may look complex to you. The fact is that people with robust, intact digestive systems can get away with eating the same foods again and again (although everyone needs to make seasonal dietary shifts in order to take in a broad range of nutrients, especially phytonutrients). But for people with digestive issues, eating too much of the same food can actually lead to a sensitivity to that food. The Gut Restoration Program is designed to mix things up with a lot of variety among the foods that are safe for you to eat. We also want to give you a lot of different types of dishes to choose from, to inspire you to be a little more adventurous, even on a limited diet.

If you truly need to reduce the amount of time you spend in the kitchen, again, it's fine to double recipes and make fewer options for each week's meals. Just be sure to rotate your staples on a weekly basis. It can work, for instance, to have smoothies every day for breakfast, or salads with simple proteins for every lunch—just make a few different types of these recipes from week to week.

◎ **Quality.** To reduce the toxic load on your system and for optimal nutrition, buy the highest-quality ingredients you can afford, such as organic produce and animal foods that are caught in the wild or raised on pasture. Fresh is best, but frozen runs a close second for nutrient content.

◎ **What to Drink.** During the twenty-eight days of the program plan to drink enough clean, filtered water to turn your urine a pale, clear yellow. That will mean different amounts of water for different people, but it probably won't be less than eight glasses per day. (Note that after taking multivitamins or other supplements containing B vitamins, urine can turn fluorescent yellow, an effect that should wear off after a couple of hours.) You can also enjoy green tea, herbal tea, unsweetened kombucha, and black tea. Remember to avoid all alcohol, cow's milk, sweetened drinks, fruit juice, and artificially flavored drinks.

◎ **Appetite.** Because there are more vegetables and fewer grains and starches than you may be used to on the Gut Restoration Program, expect your appetite to go up and down in the first week or two. If you find your appetite decreasing, it's totally fine to cut out a snack or reduce a portion size. If your appetite increases, add a snack after breakfast. If you find yourself consistently hungry after eating evening meals, it's fine to add another protein, fat, grain, or starch to your plate.

◎ **Detox Symptoms.** As you change your diet you may notice the appearance of some mild symptoms, brought on by the changes taking place in your body. For example, when you stop eating something to which you are sensitive or remove addictive foods such as sugar, you may experience a short period of discomfort. Symptoms such as mild headaches, low-grade nausea, cravings, fatigue, or emotional irritability are quite common and should go away after about three days. Once you get through this initial shift (some people don't have any difficult symptoms at all), you may see some positive signs that things are improving, such as newfound energy, glowing skin, or real relief from your digestive discomforts.

Transient Constipation

Don't be too concerned if one of your detox symptoms is a little constipation. The Gut Restoration Program is high in vegetable fiber, but low in starchy bulk from foods like bread, crackers, or beans, and for some people this may result in a few days of mild constipation. To address the issue, simply increase your water intake and know that the discomfort will pass as your body adjusts to a different way of eating.

Making Snacking Easy and Healthy

Because you are eliminating a pretty good-sized list of foods from your diet, keeping a stash of gut-friendly snacks on hand at all times will help keep you from slipping and eating foods that are not on the program. Don't expect to find fresh fruits and veggies and quality proteins when you're on the run. Shelf-stable snacks, such as nut-and-seed trail mixes and small cans of tuna or sardines, can travel anywhere—you can even keep them in your car. For fresher fare, you may want to carry a little insulated bag for cold cuts, crudités, fresh fruits, or coconut yogurt.

For IBD Sufferers (Crohn's, Ulcerative Colitis, Microscopic Colitis, etc.)

Your digestive system needs especially gentle care, so please substitute steamed or roasted greens and vegetables for raw salads and crudités in the gut-restoration meal plan and gently warm any dressing. Alternatively, if you want to incorporate some raw veggies into your diet, you can blend them into a variety of smoothies and soups to make them more digestible.

The Weekly Menus

The gut-restoration menus are divided into four one-week sections. Each week provides you with specific options for program-compliant breakfasts, lunches, dinners, and snacks for all seven days. For your convenience, there are a few instructions for advanced preparation (such as marinating meat or making Bone Broth) and suggestions for using leftovers to be used in other meals and snacks in the following days. Before creating your grocery list and shopping for the week, carefully review the week's menus and recipes, customize them to fit your needs, and plan out your food preparation strategy. Most people find it easiest to plan and shop on Saturday and spend a little time on Sunday preparing any stock items, such as salad dressing or chilled tea for smoothies, for the week to come. Every Friday night, in addition to a suggested meal, you will see options for a night out (be sure to keep your meal program-compliant!) or a "leftovers night." This is to give you a little flexibility for special plans or to use up any leftovers from the past week before shopping for the next week.

Some of the meal and snack options provide cooking or assembly instructions right in the body of the menu. Other, more complex dishes, indicated by bolded text, are broken out into actual recipes. Following the menus, you will find a listing of all the program recipes organized alphabetically in these four categories: Breakfasts, Lunches, Dinners, and Snacks and Specialty Items. Some of the recipes, such as the Basic Smoothie, Basic Bone Broth, and Basic Green Salad, are actually templates with formulas for making the dish with different ingredients. Use the ingredients suggested on the menus for the Basic Smoothie template, for example, to make a variety of different smoothies throughout the program. Before you start your program, spend a little time reviewing the menus and recipes to familiarize yourself with how the food plan works.

*NOTE: The recipe for Basic Sauerkraut (see page 164), a gut-healing dish that you can prepare at home, takes ten to fourteen days for the fermenting process to complete, so if you would like to use homemade sauerkraut for the program you will need to plan accordingly. If you don't wish to make your own from scratch, simply buy a good-quality prepared sauerkraut from the refrigerator case at your local natural foods store.

GUT RESTORATION MEAL PLAN

Meal	Breakfast	Lunch
SUN	Egg Flowers	Alaskan Salmon Salad Wraps
MON	Basic Smoothie: Green Pineapple Green tea, ½ c frozen pineapple, vanilla protein, 1 chopped celery stalk, small handful cilantro, ½" ginger root, coconut oil, stevia	Chopped leftover chicken and broccoli, black olives, sliced almonds dressed w/ 1 T each tahini and water, 2 t apple cider vinegar, and 1 t gluten-free tamari, blended
TUES	Leftover Egg Flowers	Deli-Veg Rollups
WED	Smoothie: Choco Frosty Vanilla almond milk or green tea, ½ frozen banana, choco protein, 6–7 raw Brazil nuts, 1 T cacao or cocoa powder, stevia, 5 ice cubes	Shredded leftover chicken, chopped pickles, minced red onion w/ all-natural mayo or mustard served inside hollowed-out cucumber halves
THUR	Berry Creamy Oatmeal	Simple Savory Chicken Soup w/ Chicken Bone Broth and leftover chicken
FRI	Smoothie: Wild Blues & Greens Green tea, 1 c frozen wild blueberries, dinosaur kale, vanilla protein, coconut oil, stevia, ground cinnamon	Crabacado
SAT	Apple Pancakes	Chopped salad w/ romaine, carrots, apple, and leftover diced pork dressed w/ Basic Balsamic Vinaigrette

MENU WEEK 1

Mid-Afternoon Snack	Dinner
1 apple w/ ½ T almond butter	**Pesto Chicken Thighs** w/ steamed broccoli (make extra broccoli for Mon. lunch) and baked sweet potatoes
Leftover Egg Flowers	Salmon steaks broiled w/ a light coating of Dijon mustard and dried dill, steamed artichokes w/ mayo for dipping, and **Basic Green Salad**
Roasted macadamia nuts, shaved coconut, and chopped fresh melon	2 large chickens rubbed w/ minced fresh garlic, olive oil, salt, and pepper—roasted, brown basmati rice (make a double batch of rice for Wed. dinner) and sautéed asparagus *Strip leftover meat from the chickens for leftovers, and make* **Basic Bone Broth** (Chicken)
Plain coconut yogurt w/ frozen cherries, dried coconut, dark choco chips, and stevia	**Savory Sirloin and Shiitake Salad** w/ leftover brown basmati rice *Marinate Mustard Pork Chops*
Sliced deli beef w/ a smear of leftover pesto rolled over carrot sticks	**Mustard-Marinated Pork Chops** w/ sautéed okra or steamed sweet baby peas and **Basic Green Salad**
1 piece chopped seasonal fruit with 3 T toasted sunnies or pepitas	Curried chicken salad served in lettuce cups: blend ⅔ c full-fat coconut milk, 2 pitted Medjool dates, 2 t curry powder, and salt to taste. Dress 3 c leftover chicken and chopped apple, celery, golden raisins, shredded coconut, and sliced almonds and serve in lettuce cups
1 small can tuna and ½ finely chopped fennel bulb w/ fresh-squeezed lemon juice	Leftovers, night out, or **Quick Shrimp Stir-Fry**

GUT RESTORATION MEAL PLAN

Meal	Breakfast	Lunch
SUN	**Green Pesto Egg Cups**	Deli turkey roll-ups and creamy slaw: whisk together ⅓ c prepared or leftover pesto, ¼ c all-natural mayo or coconut milk, and 2 T apple cider vinegar to dress one 10-ounce bag prepared cabbage slaw. Salt and pepper to taste. *Make Creamy Vegan Dressing.*
MON	**Smoothie: Raspberry Lime** Vanilla almond milk, 1 c raspberries, vanilla protein, zest and fruit of ½ lime, few basil leaves. Optional: stevia, avocado	Chopped romaine lettuce and leftover chicken dressed with **Creamy Vegan Dressing**
TUES	Leftover Green Pesto Egg Cups	Leftover pork tenderloin, chopped apples, chopped or steamed greens, and sliced almonds w/ drizzles of balsamic vinegar and olive oil
WED	**Smoothie: Mounds Bar** Coconut or vanilla almond milk, ½ frozen banana, 2 T shredded coconut, choco protein, cacao or cocoa, few drops stevia, avocado	Leftover creamy slaw w/ thawed frozen shrimp
THUR	**Easy Egg Drop Soup**	**Cranberry Tunacado**
FRI	**Smoothie: Choco-Orange** Choco or vanilla almond milk, fruit of 1 small naval orange w/ 1 t zest, choco protein, 2 T cacao or 1 T cocoa, 4 ice cubes, stevia, avocado	Waldorf chicken salad w/ leftover chicken: whisk together 2 T mayo or plain coconut yogurt, 2 t lemon juice, and a few drops stevia to dress leftover chicken, concord grapes, chopped romaine, apple, celery, and toasted walnuts
SAT	Scrambled eggs with nitrate-free bacon	Leftover Indian Roasted Chicken Legs w/ green salad

MENU WEEK 2

Mid-Afternoon Snack	Dinner
Plain coconut yogurt w/ chopped orange, orange zest, sprinkle of shredded coconut, and stevia	**Simple Chicken Marsala** w/ sautéed escarole and garlic, and baked winter squash
Leftover Green Pesto Egg Cups	24-ounce pork tenderloin(s) seasoned with salt, pepper, and minced garlic—roasted or grilled w/ apple sauce and leftover creamy slaw or **Basic Sauerkraut** *Marinate Teriyaki Flank Steak*
Deli turkey rolled around cucumber sticks	**Teriyaki Flank Steak** w/ brown basmati rice (make a double batch of rice for Thurs. dinner) mixed with a few T sesame seeds, and steamed green beans
Almost Instant Chocolate Protein Pudding	Chopped romaine lettuce and cucumber w/ leftover Creamy Vegan Dressing topped with cold, thinly sliced, leftover Teriyaki Flank Steak
Prepared turkey or bison jerky and juice-sweetened dried cranberries	**Chicken with Coconut Almond Sauce** w/ leftover brown basmati rice and sautéed grated zucchini
Green apple w/ 1 T almond butter	**Indian Roasted Chicken Legs** and sliced green cabbage sautéed with chopped sweet onions and apples
Snack-Size Berry Smoothie	Leftovers, night out, or **Mini-Pizzas** and **Basic Green Salad**

GUT RESTORATION MEAL PLAN

Meal	Breakfast	Lunch
SUN	**Berry Breakfast Bites**	**Tropical Shrimp Salad**
MON	**Smoothie: Thin Mint** Peppermint tea, 2 handfuls baby spinach, 1 small handful fresh mint, choco protein, cacao or cocoa, 6 Brazil nuts and/or ½ frozen banana, stevia, few ice cubes	Leftover filling from Asian Lettuce Wraps over chopped greens
TUES	**Spinach Artichoke Omelet**	Leftover tilapia, thawed frozen shrimp, or sliced deli meat over sautéed summer squash and garlic
WED	**Smoothie: Watermelon Cooler** Peppermint tea, 1 c fresh or frozen watermelon, few leaves peppermint, vanilla protein, coconut oil, stevia, few ice cubes	Chopped fresh mango, chopped avocado, and thawed frozen shrimp w/ fresh-squeezed lime juice and a drizzle of olive oil in lettuce cups
THUR	**Tropical Raw Granola** w/ a hard-boiled egg	**Alaskan Salmon Salad Wraps**
FRI	**Smoothie: Pumpkin Pie** Vanilla almond milk, ⅓ c canned pumpkin, ½ frozen banana or 2 pitted dates, ground flax, 1 t pumpkin pie spice, few drops stevia	Leftover Fruited Slow Cooker Brisket over green salad
SAT	**Pumpkin Pancakes** (w/ leftover canned pumpkin)	**Deli-Veg Rollups**

MENU WEEK 3

Mid-Afternoon Snack	Dinner
Prepared turkey or bison jerky and 1 piece fresh, seasonal fruit	**Asian Lettuce Wraps**
Leftover Berry Breakfast Bites	**Tilapia over Wilted Baby Greens** w/ baked sweet potato or winter squash
Watermelon chunks, sliced fresh mint, and toasted sliced almonds	Simple grilled sirloin steak* w/ brown basmati rice and sesame seeds, and **Basic Sauerkraut** (*Make 2–3 extra steaks for tomorrow's dinner and a double batch of rice for Thurs. dinner)
2 parts plain coconut yogurt mixed w/ 1 part canned pumpkin, pumpkin pie spice, and stevia	**Kicky Steak Salad** w/ leftover sirloin
Snack-Size Berry Smoothie	**Fruited Slow Cooker Brisket** over leftover brown basmati rice and roasted Brussels sprouts
Almost Instant Chocolate Protein Pudding	**Coconut Shrimp** w/ tropical quinoa (replace half the water with light coconut milk and stir in baby spinach and finely chopped pineapple once off the heat)
Chopped boiled egg w/ chopped celery, mayo, or coconut yogurt and pinches of curry powder, salt, and pepper in lettuce wraps	Leftovers, night out, or **Satisfying Bacon-Stuffed Sweet Potatoes** and **Basic Green Salad**

GUT RESTORATION MEAL PLAN

Meal	Breakfast	Lunch
SUN	**Egg and Portobello Florentine**	**Citrus Shrimp Salad**
MON	**Smoothie: Green Pineapple** Coconut or vanilla almond milk, ½ c frozen pineapple, vanilla protein, 1 chopped celery stalk, small handful cilantro, ½" ginger root, coconut oil, and stevia	Leftover Mango Meatloaf Muffins w/ steamed broccoli
TUES	**Perfect Minute Omelet** w/ chopped seasonal fruit	Leftover Flank Steak over chopped greens and cucumber with drizzles of sesame oil and rice vinegar
WED	**Smoothie: Carrot Cake** Coconut or vanilla almond milk, ¼ c pineapple, 1 small carrot, chopped (steam first if you don't have an industrial blender), vanilla protein, 1 T shredded coconut, coconut oil, stevia, and 1 t orange zest, optional walnuts, cinnamon, ginger, and dash of nutmeg	Leftover Pesto Chicken Thighs w/ sautéed asparagus
THUR	**Easy Egg Drop Soup**	**Crabacado** w/ cherry tomatoes
FRI	**Smoothie: Choco-Orange** Coconut, vanilla, or choco almond milk, fruit of 1 small naval orange w/ 1 t zest, choco protein, 2 T cacao or 1 T cocoa, 4 ice cubes, avocado, and stevia	Leftover Chicken and Wild Rice Soup and salad
SAT	**Berry Creamy Oatmeal**	Leftover lamb chops and green salad

MENU WEEK 4

Mid-Afternoon Snack	Dinner
Tangy Lemon Oat Bars	**Mango Meatloaf Muffins** w/ steamed green beans and **Basic Green Salad** *Marinate Teriyaki Flank Steak*
Chopped boiled egg and deli turkey, sprouts or shredded carrots, and all-natural mayo or mustard rolled up in romaine leaves	**Teriyaki Flank Steak** w/ brown rice and sesame seeds (make extra rice for Sushi Salad recipe Wed. night) w/ steamed greens
Leftover Tangy Lemon Oat Bars	**Pesto Chicken Thighs** w/ steamed artichokes and sautéed summer squash
Spinach apple soup: 2 c baby spinach blended with small peeled and chopped apple, ¼ c raw cashews or avocado, ⅔ c water, salt, and pepper, to taste	**Sushi Salad**
Plain coconut yogurt w/ shaved coconut, sliced almonds, lime zest and juice, and a few drops stevia	**Chicken and Wild Rice Soup** w/ **Basic Green Salad** *Herb-Marinate Lamb Chops*
Roasted almonds, dried or fresh tart cherries, and dark chocolate chips	**Herb-Marinated Lamb Chops** w/ roasted beets and sautéed greens
Creamy Frozen Fruit	Leftovers, night out or **Greek Frittata** with steamed broccoli

Mindful Eating for Improved Digestion

When your body is in stress mode, digestion takes a backseat to other physiological processes. (See page 46 for a thorough discussion of the effect stress has on the gut.) Eating meals while feeling tense is a setup for continuing digestive woes, while eating in a relaxed state optimizes the natural processes of digestion. Bringing some conscious awareness into the largely automatic habit of eating has a calming effect on both the mind and the body and a beneficial effect on digestion. Use these guidelines to help you be more mindful whenever you sit down to eat:

Hunger Cues

- Hollow feeling near solar plexus
- Stomach "growling" above the belt line
- Light shakiness or mild lightheadedness
- Overall sense of emptiness or hunger

When possible, find or create surroundings that are soothing to your mind and pleasing to your senses.

Eat when your body is actually hungry, not out of habit or to soothe an uncomfortable emotional state

When you eat, only eat. (Don't mix eating with other activities, including watching TV, texting, or driving.)

Before tasting your first mouthful of food, take a few moments to just notice your emotional state and draw in a few deep breaths. Just that touch of awareness and three to five deep breaths will help to "digest" and calm any tension you are feeling.

Express gratitude for your food and its source.

"Taste" the food with your other senses (use your eyes, nose, ears, fingers) before you put it into your mouth. Pay attention to the food's aromas, flavors, and textures, and savor them as you eat.

Chew each bite thoroughly, especially carbohydrates. Try to break the food down completely into liquid and pulp, usually fifteen to twenty-five chews per bite. (See page 3 for tips on chewing your food.)

Pause between mouthfuls.

Remember to check your hunger and satisfaction levels every few bites.

Slow down eating as your hunger diminishes and stop when you are satisfied, but not completely full.

Satiety (Satisfaction) Cues:
- Gentle pressure or weight near solar plexus
- Reduction of food's taste appeal as the meal goes on
- Sense of peacefulness or relaxation
- Overall sense of being gently energized

Rest quietly for a few minutes after eating before you get up from the table.

The Recipes

The recipes in the Gut Restoration Program, indicated by bolded text in the menus, are listed alphabetically under *Breakfasts, Lunches, Dinners, Snacks and Specialty Items.* Be sure to note on the menu whether you should make extra side dishes for leftovers you can eat later in the week. Enjoy!

Breakfasts

Apple or Pumpkin Pancakes

1 serving

	olive oil or nut oil spray
1	egg and 1 egg white
¼	cup pumpkin puree or grated apple (unpeeled)
3	tablespoons ground flaxseed
1	packet stevia (or a few drops liquid stevia), or to taste
½	teaspoon pumpkin pie spice
½	teaspoon cinnamon
	Pinch of salt

Spray a nonstick skillet lightly with olive or nut oil and heat over medium.

In a small bowl, whisk the eggs well. Add the pumpkin puree, flaxseed, stevia, spices, and salt and whisk until smooth.

When the pan is hot, pour the batter evenly into one or two round pancakes (it will be runny) and do not disturb for about 2 minutes. Cover the pan and continue cooking until the bottoms of the cakes have browned and they are holding together well.

Carefully flip them once and cook, uncovered, for just a few minutes until the other side is nicely browned. Serve immediately.

Basic Smoothie

1 serving

For the Liquid Base

1 cup unsweetened almond milk, unsweetened coconut milk (in a carton, not canned), coconut water, chilled tea, or water*

Fruit and Vegetables

½–1 cup chopped fruit (berries, melon, peaches, pineapple, mango, orange, lemon, lime, etc.) or vegetables (celery, carrot, pumpkin, sweet potato, etc.) in amounts indicated on the menus or to taste. Steam or bake veggies before use for more digestive ease.

Protein

1 scoop unsweetened vegan protein powder (hemp, rice, or a combination—avoid soy— menu plan calls for both vanilla and chocolate)

Extra Fiber

2 tablespoons seeds (ground flax, hemp hearts), optional if adding greens or extra nuts/seeds

Fat

1 tablespoon oil (flax, hemp, coconut, Omega 3-6-9) or ¼ ripe Hass avocado

Optional Additions

1 large handful leafy greens (try baby spinach, stemmed dinosaur kale, etc.)

1 small handful fresh herbs (try cilantro, parsley, mint, etc.)

1	tablespoon raw cacao or cocoa powder, nuts, seeds or nut/seed butters, gluten-free rolled oats, grated fresh ginger, citrus juice, or 1 teaspoon greens powder, etc.
½–1	teaspoon optional spices (citrus zest, cinnamon, ground ginger, etc.) or a thumb-sized chunk of ginger root
	Few drops liquid stevia, 1–2 pitted dates, ¼ frozen banana, etc. as sweeteners

Combine all ingredients according to the menu plan except fat in an industrial-strength blender (such as Vitamix, Ninja, or Nutribullet) and blend until smooth. Add fat of choice and blend briefly to incorporate. Add 3–6 ice cubes for a frostier smoothie.

*You can usually use these liquids interchangeably for the liquid base. The tea option will be lighter than the almond milk, and almond milk will be lighter than the coconut milk, so plan accordingly for your hunger needs.

To make chilled tea, place 3 tea bags in a 1-quart Mason jar and fill with boiling water. Cover and let steep for 10 minutes, remove tea bags, and chill tea in the refrigerator for smoothie use all week. Sundays are a great day to make your cold tea base.

Berry Breakfast Bites

16 Berry Bites, 3-4 servings

3   soft Medjool dates, pitted (or 4 regular, pitted)

1   cup raw cashews

¼   cup almond butter

¼   cup shredded coconut

1   scoop vanilla protein powder

    Few drops vanilla stevia, optional, to taste

3   tablespoons coconut oil, melted, but not hot

½   cup blueberries, fresh or frozen, no need to thaw (or other berries, chopped if large)

Combine all ingredients from dates through coconut oil in a food processor. Process steadily until well combined and holding together in a dough, about a minute. Fold in blueberries and, using your hands, shape dough into 16 balls (about 2 inches in diameter). Berry Bites will keep for about 3 days in the fridge. Enjoy.

Berry Creamy Oatmeal

1 serving

1	cup unsweetened vanilla almond milk
1	egg
½	cup whole-rolled gluten-free oats
	Pinch of salt
⅓	cup sliced berries (fresh or frozen), or any chopped seasonal fruit
½	teaspoon cinnamon
1	teaspoon coconut nectar or few drops liquid stevia, to taste
1	teaspoon vanilla
2	tablespoons almond slices

In a small saucepan, whisk together the milk and egg and mix in the oats and salt over medium heat. Bring to a low boil over medium heat, continuing to whisk frequently. Reduce heat and cook for about 10 minutes or until the oats are tender, whisking frequently. In the last minute of cooking time, mix the berries and cinnamon into the oatmeal. Stir in sweetener, vanilla, and almonds just before serving.

Easy Egg Drop Soup

1 serving

2 cups chicken bone broth (see recipe for Basic Bone Broth on page 160)

1+ cups bite-sized mixed frozen vegetables* (corn, carrots, broccoli, mushrooms, spinach, pearl onions, etc.)

2 eggs, lightly beaten

Salt and pepper, to taste (or low-sodium, gluten-free tamari or coconut aminos**)

2 tablespoons chopped fresh scallions, chives, cilantro, or basil

Heat the broth in a medium saucepan over high heat. Add the frozen veggies and cook for 2–3 minutes until tender. Slowly pour the eggs into the boiling soup and stir for about a minute or until the eggs are cooked and swirled around the soup. Remove from heat, top with herbs, and serve immediately.

*You can also use fresh or leftover cooked veggies in this recipe—simply adjust the cooking time as necessary before adding the eggs. Leftover roasted greens work nicely in this recipe as well.

**Coconut aminos are a gluten- and soy-free alternative to soy sauce. They are not as salty as soy sauce or tamari but have a very similar flavor profile. Look for coconut aminos in natural food stores.

Egg and Portobello Florentine

4 servings

High-heat cooking oil spray

4 large portobello mushroom caps, stemmed, and gills removed*

1 tablespoon olive oil

2 cloves garlic, minced

1 10-ounce bag baby spinach

1 10-ounce bag baby arugula

Salt and freshly ground pepper, to taste

½ teaspoon salt (can omit if eggs** are very fresh)

1 teaspoon apple cider vinegar (can omit if eggs** are very fresh)

4 very fresh, extra-large eggs

½ large, ripe Hass avocado, sliced thinly, optional

8 teaspoons prepared dairy-free pesto (or see page 163 for Basic Dairy-Free Pesto recipe), or to taste

Preheat the broiler and lightly spray a broiler pan with high-heat cooking oil. Place the prepared portobellos top-down on the broiler pan and broil for about 7–8 minutes or until tender—watch closely to prevent burning.

While the mushrooms are cooking, heat the oil in a large sauté pan. Add spinach and arugula, and cover for 1 minute to wilt slightly. Remove the cover, season with salt and pepper to taste, turn gently for even cooking, and continue to sauté for another 2 minutes or until the greens are wilted to desired tenderness.

While the greens are wilting, fill a medium sauté pan about half-full of water, add salt and vinegar, if using, and bring the water just to a simmer

THE MEAL PLAN AND RECIPES

(not a full boil!). Break the eggs one at a time into a small bowl and slide them gently into the simmering water. Try to slide them against the edge of the sauté pan to help them keep their shape. Simmer the eggs for about 4 minutes or until the whites are cooked through but the yolks are still soft. Using a slotted spoon, remove the eggs from the pan and set them aside to drain.

While the eggs are draining, place one broiled portobello cap on each of 4 plates. Lay ¼ of the avocado slices, if using, evenly over each mushroom, and top with ¼ of the prepared greens and 1 poached egg. Spoon 2 teaspoons of pesto (or to taste) over the egg and serve immediately.

*To stem the portobellos, gently pinch and grip the stem firmly at the base with one hand, and slowly twist the cap with the other hand until the stem separates. To remove the gills, scoop them out with a teaspoon, leaving hollowed-out shells.

**The freshest eggs have very firm whites and yolks, so they tend to retain their shape better when cooking. If you didn't buy your eggs at a farm stand, use the salt and vinegar to help them hold their shape when poaching.

Egg Flowers

6 egg flowers, 3 servings

Olive oil spray

6 (or more) slices organic deli ham or turkey

6 (or more) pastured eggs

Salt and pepper, to taste

Extras (optional)

Chopped olives, Italian seasoning, curry powder or cooked veggies such as mushrooms, carrots, peppers, onions, broccoli, etc.

Set the oven to 350°F.

Lightly spray the cups of a 6-cup muffin pan with oil and gently fold one slice of deli meat into each cup. Crack one egg into each cup and season to taste with salt and pepper. Top with a sprinkle of any optional extras, and bake for about 18 minutes or until eggs are just cooked through.

Greek Frittata

4 servings

8	eggs
⅔	cup unsweetened plain almond milk
1	teaspoon oregano
¼	cup fresh basil, slivered (or 2 teaspoons dried)
½	teaspoon each salt and freshly ground pepper
2	tablespoons olive oil
2	cloves garlic, minced
2	cups baby spinach
1	14-ounce can artichoke hearts in water, well drained and coarsely chopped
½	cup sliced and pitted kalamata olives

Preheat oven to broil.

In a large bowl, combine the eggs, almond milk, oregano, basil, and salt and pepper, and whisk until beaten. Set aside.

Smooth the oil over the entire surface of a 10-inch cast iron skillet to lightly coat and heat over medium. Add the garlic, spinach, artichoke hearts, and olives. Cover and cook for 2 minutes or until spinach is wilted. Remove cover, stir the vegetables, and pour the beaten eggs over them. Cook for about 5 minutes or until the outer edge is cooked but the center is still unset. Put the pan under the broiler for about 3-4 minutes or until the center is set and the surface has begun to brown, watching carefully to prevent overcooking.

Green Pesto Egg Cups

6 egg cups, 3 servings

1   packed cup arugula, stemmed collard greens, or spinach

¼   cup prepared pesto (or chopped kalamata olives) (see page 163 for Basic Dairy-Free Pesto Recipe)

5   eggs

Salt and freshly ground pepper, to taste

⅓   ripe avocado, finely diced, optional

Preheat the oven to 350°F.

Line a muffin tin with 6 parchment muffin cups and set aside.

Pulse the greens in a food processor (or chop by hand) until finely chopped but not pureed, scraping down the sides as necessary. Remove the blade and stir in the pesto.

In a medium bowl, whisk the eggs, salt, and pepper until just blended. Add the prepared vegetables and avocado, if using, and mix gently to combine well. Spoon about ¼ cup of the mixture into each of the muffin cups and bake for 18–20 minutes or until the egg is set and just-dry on top.

Perfect Minute Omelet

1 serving

2 eggs

1 tablespoon water

Pinch of salt

Pinch of freshly ground pepper

1 teaspoon coconut oil

Lightly whisk the eggs, water, salt and pepper together in a small bowl and set aside.

Heat the coconut oil in a small sauté or omelet pan (7–8-inches) over high heat, swirling to coat the pan for about 1 minute or until the coconut oil is fully melted and distributed evenly across the bottom and sides of the pan. When the pan is well coated and hot, pour the eggs into the pan and do not disturb for about 30 seconds. When eggs are bubbling and the bottom surface has solidified, gently lift one half of the omelet and fold it over the other half. Let it cook for another 20 seconds or until desired doneness and slide it out onto your plate. If you prefer your eggs to be well cooked, you may flip the omelet over and cook for another 10–20 seconds before plating.

Spinach Artichoke Omelet

1 serving

2	eggs
1	tablespoon water
½	teaspoon each salt and freshly ground pepper
2	teaspoons olive oil
¾	cup baby spinach
2	marinated artichoke hearts, drained and finely chopped

Combine the eggs, water, salt, and pepper in a small bowl and whisk until lightly beaten. Set aside.

Heat the olive oil in a 12-inch non stick skillet over medium heat. Add the spinach and cover for 1 minute. Increase the heat to medium high for 1 minute and sprinkle the artichoke hearts over the spinach. Pour the eggs evenly over the spinach and artichoke hearts and let the mixture sit undisturbed for 1 minute. Working gently, lift one half of the omelet and flip it over the other half. Cook for about 30 seconds and flip once to cook to desired doneness.

Tropical Raw Granola

1 serving

About	7 almonds
About	5 macadamia nuts
⅓	cup light coconut milk
¼	teaspoon vanilla stevia
3	tablespoons whole-rolled, gluten-free oats
2	tablespoons finely chopped pineapple or mango, optional
1	tablespoon shredded coconut (or 2 teaspoons grated)
½	teaspoon lime zest, optional

Combine the almonds, macadamia nuts, coconut milk, and stevia in a food processor and pulse until the nuts are the size of coarse crumbs—don't overprocess. Transfer mixture to a small bowl and stir in oats, fruit, if using, shredded coconut, and lime zest, if using. Serve at room temperature, or warm the mixture for a few minutes in a small saucepan over low heat.

Lunches

Alaskan Salmon Salad Wraps

1 generous serving

2	tablespoons olive oil
	Juice and zest of ½ small lemon
2	teaspoons red wine vinegar
1	teaspoon Dijon mustard
½	teaspoon oregano
¼	teaspoon each garlic and onion powder, optional
	Salt and freshly ground pepper, to taste
1	4-ounce can wild Alaskan salmon, skin and bones removed
1	loosely packed cup mild sprouts, any variety
1–2	tablespoons finely chopped red onion, to taste
5	kalamata olives, pitted and chopped
2	artichoke hearts canned in water, drained and chopped, optional
4	large romaine leaves

In a medium bowl whisk together the olive oil, lemon juice and zest, red wine vinegar, Dijon mustard, oregano, garlic and onion powders if using, salt, and pepper. Add the salmon, sprouts, red onion, and olives, and mix thoroughly with a fork. Fold in the artichoke hearts, if using, and divide the salad evenly among the lettuce leaves and serve.

Citrus Shrimp Salad

1 generous serving

For the Dressing

Juice from ½ large naval orange

1   teaspoon orange zest

Juice from ½ lemon

1   ¾-inch knob of peeled ginger, chopped

Few drops stevia, to taste

Pinch of sea salt

For the Salad

½   cup grated jicama (or carrot)

1   cup baby spinach

1   cup baby arugula (or double spinach)

1   pink grapefruit, supreme cut (segments cut
     from the membrane and pith)

⅓   avocado, chopped

6-8   large cooked, chilled shrimp

¼   cup chopped cilantro, optional

2-3   tablespoons crushed macadamia nuts

Combine all dressing ingredients in an immersion blender and blend until smooth. Taste and adjust seasonings if necessary.

Pour a couple of tablespoons of the dressing over the jicama in a small bowl and toss to coat. Let marinate for a few minutes or while preparing the rest of the salad. In a large salad bowl, combine all remaining salad ingredients from spinach through cilantro. Add the jicama and just enough additional dressing to coat everything lightly. Toss well to combine and top with the macadamia nuts. Serve immediately.

NOTE: If you don't have an immersion blender, either grate or finely mince the ginger root or substitute ½ teaspoon ground ginger and whisk ingredients together.

Crabacado

1 serving

1	tablespoon plain coconut yogurt or all-natural mayonnaise
	Generous squeeze lemon juice
	Pinch of salt
1-2	tablespoons chopped fresh cilantro or green onion, optional
1	6-ounce can lump crabmeat, well drained
½	ripe Hass avocado, peeled and pitted

In a small bowl, whisk together the coconut yogurt or mayonnaise, lemon juice, salt, and herbs until well combined. Gently stir in crabmeat until well coated. Mound crab salad evenly over the avocado and serve.

Cranberry Tunacado

1 serving

2   tablespoons all-natural mayonnaise

3   tablespoons finely chopped celery

1   tablespoon juice-sweetened dried
    cranberries

1   tablespoon toasted sliced almonds

1   4- or 5-ounce can water-packed tuna,
    drained

½   ripe Hass avocado, peeled and pitted

In a medium bowl combine the mayonnaise, celery, cranberries, and almonds and mix to combine. Add the tuna and flake it apart. Mix to combine. Spoon the tuna mixture over the avocado and serve.

Deli-Veg Rollups

1 serving

1   cup packed baby spinach

½   crisp red apple, unpeeled, seeded, and roughly chopped

1-2 teaspoons seasoning of your choice (try prepared horseradish or finely minced fresh ginger or fresh-squeezed lemon juice or Dijon mustard)

6   thin slices high-quality deli roast beef, ham, or turkey

½   small ripe Hass avocado, peeled, and mashed into a paste

Combine the spinach and apple in a food processor and pulse until finely chopped but not pureed, scraping down the sides as necessary. Stir in the seasoning of your choice. Double up the deli slices and lay out to form 3 "wraps." Spread equal amounts of the avocado onto each wrap. Spoon equal portions of the spinach and apple mixture over the avocado, roll up the wraps as tightly as cigars, serve immediately.

Simple Savory Chicken Soup

1 serving

2	cups chicken bone broth or no-sodium broth or water (see page 160 for Basic Bone Broth recipe)
1	teaspoon turmeric, optional
1	teaspoon onion powder, optional
1	cup finely chopped fresh or frozen seasonal vegetables (sweet onion, carrots, leafy greens, broccoli, peas, sweet potato, winter squash, etc.)
1–2	tablespoons rice miso, to taste (or low-sodium, gluten-free tamari)
⅔	cup shredded cooked chicken

Combine the broth, turmeric, and onion powder, if using, and bring to a boil over high heat in a medium saucepan. Reduce heat to medium and add the vegetables, simmering for about 4 minutes or to desired tenderness. Add the chicken and cook for about 1 minute until warm. Remove soup from heat and gently whisk in the miso* until incorporated. Serve immediately.

*To blend the miso perfectly into your soup, put the paste into a small bowl, then gradually add ¼ cup of the hot broth. Whisk the paste into the liquid to blend it in thoroughly, then pour the mixture back into the saucepan and mix it gently into the rest of the soup.

Tropical Shrimp Salad

1 serving

2	tablespoons coconut milk
2	tablespoons diced ripe mango
¼	teaspoon curry powder
	Pinch of salt
2	tablespoons chopped cilantro
¼	teaspoon brown mustard seeds, optional
1	cup sliced Napa cabbage (or hardy lettuce)
¼	ripe Hass avocado, peeled and sliced
4	ounces cooked shrimp, peeled and deveined*
1	teaspoons dried or shaved coconut, optional

Combine the coconut milk, mango, curry powder, and salt in a mini-blender (or use an immersion blender) and blend until smooth. Stir in the cilantro and mustard seeds, if using, and set aside. To serve, arrange the cabbage and avocado slices on a plate and top with the shrimp. Drizzle the coconut mango cream over the top and sprinkle with the coconut, if using.

*You may also sauté or grill raw shrimp, rubbed with salt and curry powder, if you'd prefer them hot.

Dinners

Asian Lettuce Wraps

4 servings plus extra for lunch

1½	tablespoons sesame oil
4	ounces sliced shitake caps, finely chopped
4	large garlic cloves, minced
1	8-ounce can of sliced water chestnuts, finely chopped
1½	pounds leanest ground turkey (or leanest ground beef)
½	teaspoon salt
3	tablespoons low-sodium, gluten-free tamari
3	tablespoons mirin*
2	teaspoons toasted sesame oil
1	cup sliced green onion (greens only)
2	cups mung bean sprouts (or shredded Napa cabbage or lettuce)
1	head large-leaf lettuce, cored and separated into leaves

In a large skillet, heat the oil over medium high. Add the shitakes and garlic and cook for 2 minutes. Add the water chestnuts, turkey, and salt and sauté for about 5 minutes or until almost no pink remains, draining any excess oil if necessary. Stir the tamari and mirin into the turkey, and continue to cook until the turkey is cooked through and all the vegetables are hot, about 3 minutes. Remove from heat and stir in sesame oil, green onions, and bean sprouts. Serve with lettuce leaves for scooping or wrapping.

*Mirin is a Japanese sweet wine condiment.

Chicken and Wild Rice Soup

about 5 servings (set aside 1 serving for lunch)

2	tablespoons olive oil
3	large shallots, chopped (or 1 small yellow onion, chopped)
3	medium carrots, peeled and cut into ½-inch rounds
6	cups chicken broth (see page 160 for Bone Broth recipe)
⅓	cup uncooked wild rice
1	large sweet potato, peeled and chopped
2	large boneless, skinless chicken breasts, sliced into bite-sized pieces (or 2 pounds chicken tenders)
1	cup frozen corn
2	tablespoons mirin**
½	teaspoon tarragon
¼	teaspoon thyme
¾	teaspoon salt
½	teaspoon pepper
⅓	cup golden raisins (or regular or dried cranberries)

In a large soup pot, heat olive oil over medium heat. Add shallots and sauté for 3 minutes. Add carrots and sauté for another 3 minutes. Pour broth over all, increase heat to high, and bring soup to a low boil. Add wild rice and sweet potato. Lower heat and simmer, covered, for 20 minutes. Stir in chicken and cook for 10 minutes. Stir in mirin, tarragon, thyme, salt, pepper, and raisins. Simmer for 10 minutes until rice and chicken are cooked through.

**Mirin is a Japanese sweet wine condiment available in Asian markets, natural food stores, or the ethnic food sections of large grocery chains.

Coconut Shrimp

about 4 servings

For the Shrimp

⅔ cup raw macadamia nuts

2 teaspoons palm sugar or erythritol*

1 teaspoon onion powder

½ teaspoon salt

2 extra-large eggs

¾ cup unsweetened shredded coconut

1 pound large raw shrimp, cleaned, shelled, deveined except for tails, and butterflied

For the Coconut Mango Dip (optional)

⅔ packed cup diced fresh ripe mango

⅓ cup light coconut milk (or plain coconut yogurt)

Juice of ½ small lime

Pinch of salt

Few drops liquid stevia, to taste

Place rack in the middle of the oven and preheat to 425°F.

Line a large baking sheet with parchment paper and set aside. Combine the macadamia nuts, palm sugar, onion powder, and salt in a food processor and pulse into fine crumbs. Do not overprocess or the nuts will become oily. Transfer the nut mix into a shallow dish for dipping.

In another shallow bowl, beat the eggs.

Place the coconut in a third shallow dish. Holding the shrimp by their tails, dip them first into the beaten egg and shake off any excess. Then dip them lightly into the nut mix to coat, then redip them lightly in the beaten egg and roll them in the coconut. Gently lay the shrimp on the prepared baking sheet and repeat until all shrimp are coated. Bake, turning the shrimp once halfway through cook time, for 15 minutes or until coconut is lightly golden.

To make the dipping sauce, combine all ingredients from mango through stevia into the cup for an immersion blender or into a small blender and blend until smooth. Taste and adjust for tanginess and sweetness if necessary. Serve shrimp with sauce on the side, if using.

*Erythritol is a granulated low-glycemic sweetener that is available in natural food stores. You can also find it in regular supermarket chains under the brand name Truvia.

Fruited Slow Cooker Brisket

about 6 servings (set aside 2 servings for lunch)

1	large sweet onion, thickly chopped
1	cup whole pitted prunes
½	cup whole dried apricots
1	4–5 pound beef brisket, sliced in half if necessary to fit into slow cooker
	Salt and pepper, to taste
¾	cup good red wine
¼	cup balsamic vinegar

Spread the onion and a few of the dried fruits evenly over the bottom of a slow cooker. Cut away any large areas of fat from the brisket with a sharp knife, season to taste with salt and pepper, and lay it over the onions and fruit, fat side up (note, removing too much of the fat will reduce the cooking time, sometimes significantly).

In a small bowl, combine the wine and vinegar. Scatter the last half of the dried fruits on top of the brisket and pour the wine/vinegar mixture lightly over the brisket. Make sure that most of the fruits stay on top of the meat to prevent them from breaking down in the liquids. Cook for 4–6 hours on high or 5–8 hours on low or until meat is cooked through and falling apart, but not dried out. Carefully remove the brisket and shred with two forks. Spoon the onions and fruit out of the liquid—they will be falling-apart soft—top each serving of brisket with a spoonful and serve.

NOTE: Slow-cooking the wine will evaporate the alcohol content.

Herb-Marinated Lamb Chops

5 servings (set aside 1 serving for lunch)

¼	cup low-sodium, gluten-free tamari
3	tablespoons olive oil
	Juice of 1 large lemon
¾	teaspoon freshly ground pepper
½	teaspoon salt
4	cloves garlic, minced
⅓	cup mint leaves, chopped
¼	cup fresh rosemary leaves, chopped
3	tablespoons fresh thyme leaves, chopped
5	lamb blade chops

In a shallow glass storage container, whisk together the tamari, olive oil, lemon juice, pepper, and salt. Add garlic, mint, rosemary, and thyme, and mix thoroughly.

Lay the lamb chops in a single layer in the dish and flip a few times to coat with the herbs and marinade. Cover and marinate for 30 minutes to overnight, flipping several times (the longer the marinating time, the more flavorful the chops). Grill the chops over medium heat for about for 6–7 minutes, flip, and grill for 4–5 minutes more for medium rare or to desired doneness.

Indian Roasted Chicken Legs

about 5 servings (set aside 1 serving for lunch)

¼	cup coconut oil, melted
2	tablespoons all-natural mayonnaise
1	tablespoon Dijon mustard
1½	tablespoons ground garam masala
1	teaspoon sea salt
	Freshly ground pepper, to taste
10–12	chicken legs

Preheat oven to 425°F.

In a small bowl, combine the oil, mayonnaise, mustard, garam masala, salt, and pepper and whisk to form a smooth sauce. Pat the chicken pieces dry and arrange in a roasting pan. Generously brush the tops and sides of each chicken leg with equal parts of the sauce. Roast for 35–40 minutes or until golden brown and cooked through.

Kicky Steak Salad

4 servings

For the Dressing

¼   cup prepared horseradish, or to taste

2   tablespoons all-natural mayonnaise or plain coconut yogurt

1   tablespoon Dijon mustard, or to taste

1   tablespoon raw apple cider vinegar

¼   teaspoon each salt and freshly ground pepper

¼   cup olive oil

For the Salad

6   cups mixed salad greens

1½   cups diced cucumbers

½   cup grated carrots

3   green onions, thinly sliced, optional

1   pound grilled sirloin steak, sliced thinly

In a small bowl, whisk together the horseradish, mayonnaise or plain coconut yogurt, Dijon mustard, vinegar, salt, and pepper until well combined. Whisk in the olive oil. Taste and adjust the seasonings if necessary. Set aside.

In a large bowl combine the salad greens, cucumber, carrots, green onion, if using, and dress to taste. Toss gently until well coated. Plate 4 equal salads and top with equal portions of the sliced steak. Drizzle a little dressing over the meat and serve.

Mango Meatloaf Muffins

12 muffins

Olive oil cooking spray

1 egg

½ cup prepared mango chutney, or to taste (any type of fruit-based chutney can be used)

1½ pounds leanest ground turkey

¼ cup whole-rolled, gluten-free oats (or 3 tablespoons ground flaxseed)

1 cup grated carrots

1 teaspoon mustard powder

1 teaspoon onion powder

1 teaspoon cracked black pepper

¾ teaspoon salt

Preheat oven to 375°F.

Lightly spray a 12-cup muffin pan with cooking oil. In a large bowl, whisk together the egg and chutney. Add turkey, oats, carrots, mustard powder, onion powder, pepper, and salt and mix gently with your hands just until combined. Spoon the mixture gently and evenly into 12 muffin cups (do not pack it in). Bake for about 30 minutes or until cooked through.

Mini-Pizzas

4 servings

For the Crust

3   cups almond flour

1   tablespoon Italian seasoning

1   teaspoon salt

½   teaspoon baking soda

3   eggs

3   tablespoons olive oil

For the Topping

3   cups organic sweet corn kernels, thawed
     if frozen

1   cup baby arugula or fresh basil

3   tablespoons pine nuts

¼–½ teaspoon each salt and freshly ground
     pepper, to taste

3   tablespoons olive oil

8   ounces cooked ham, turkey, chicken, or
     shrimp, chopped or shredded (you can use
     high-quality deli meats, but in that case you
     may want to omit the salt in the topping)

Preheat the oven to 350°F.

Cover a large baking sheet with parchment paper and set aside.

Place all crust ingredients from almond flour through olive oil in order printed from top to bottom in a food processor and pulse until just mixed and dough is holding together. Divide the dough into 4 equal parts and roll into loose balls. Arrange them evenly on a prepared baking sheet. Using your fingers or an oiled rolling pin, spread the batter into circles about 6 inches in diameter or 4 x 5-inch rectangles, about ¼-inch thick. Bake for 15 minutes.

While the crust is baking, combine the topping ingredients from corn kernels through salt and pepper in a clean food processor and pulse until the topping is mixed but still chunky—do not overprocess. Add the oil and pulse a couple of times to incorporate. Set aside.

Remove the crusts from the oven and top each mini-pizza with ¼ of the corn pesto and 2 ounces of your protein of choice. Return to the oven and warm for 2–3 minutes.

Chicken with Coconut Almond Sauce

5 servings (set aside 1 serving for lunch)

¼	cup almond butter
¼	cup coconut milk*
2	tablespoons fresh-squeezed lime juice
2	tablespoons water
2	teaspoons low-sodium, gluten-free tamari
2	teaspoons coconut nectar
½	teaspoon onion powder, optional
	Salt and freshly ground pepper, to taste
5	boneless chicken breasts**
	Sprinkles of salt and freshly ground pepper, to taste
⅓	cup chopped fresh cilantro, optional

Preheat grill to medium.

Combine the almond butter, coconut milk, lime juice, water, tamari, coconut nectar, onion powder if using, salt, and pepper and blend with an immersion blender or in a mini-blender until smooth. Set aside for the flavors to meld.

Season the chicken breasts to taste with salt and pepper. Place the chicken on the hottest part of the grill and leave undisturbed for 4–5 minutes until it is becoming opaque. Flip and cook it for another 4–5 minutes until just cooked through. Allow the chicken to rest for a couple of minutes before serving. Top generously with sauce, garnish with cilantro, if using, and serve.

*If you don't have any open coconut milk to use and have to break into a new can, pour the remainder into an ice cube tray and freeze for use in your smoothies. You may also use the coconut milk from a carton, but your sauce won't taste as rich.

**For more even grilling, pound the raw chicken breasts between two sheets of wax paper with a meat mallet to an even thickness before seasoning.

Mustard-Marinated Pork Chops

5–6 servings (set aside 2 servings for lunches)

4–6	boneless pork chops, about 1 inch thick, trimmed
	Sea salt and pepper, to taste
⅓	cup Dijon mustard
3	tablespoons coconut nectar
2	tablespoons apple cider vinegar
2	tablespoons olive oil
4	garlic cloves, minced
	Sea salt and freshly ground pepper to taste

Preheat oven to 350°F.

Lightly season the pork chops with salt and pepper and arrange them in a single layer in a shallow glass baking dish. Set aside.

Combine the mustard, coconut nectar, vinegar, and olive oil in a small bowl and whisk until smooth (or use an immersion blender). Stir in garlic and spread evenly over the pork, turning to thoroughly coat each piece. Cover and refrigerate for 6 hours to overnight.

Transfer the baking dish to the oven and cook the pork chops for 15 minutes in the marinade. Flip the chops and continue baking them for 10–15 minutes, or until an instant-read thermometer inserted into the thickest part of the meat reads 155°F. Transfer the pork chops to a platter and serve with a small amount of the pan sauce.

Pesto Chicken Thighs

about 5 servings (set aside 1 serving for lunch)

2½	pounds boneless, skinless chicken thighs (about 10)
½	cup plus 2 tablespoons prepared vegan pesto or see page 163 for Basic Dairy-Free Pesto recipe

Preheat the oven to 350°F.

Arrange the chicken thighs in a single layer in an 11 x 7-inch baking pan. Spoon ½ cup of the pesto over the top and distribute it evenly over the chicken with a butter knife. Bake for 25–35 minutes until the chicken thighs are cooked through and juicy. Toss the hot chicken with 2 tablespoons of the fresh pesto just before serving.

Quick Shrimp Stir-Fry

4 servings

1½	tablespoons sesame oil
3	cloves garlic, minced
3	tablespoons grated fresh ginger
1	pound medium shrimp, peeled and deveined (fresh or frozen, thawed)
1	12-ounce bag fresh slaw mix (shredded cabbage, carrots, and broccoli)
1	tablespoon mirin*
2	tablespoons low-sodium, gluten-free tamari
2	teaspoons toasted sesame oil, optional
1	tablespoon toasted sesame seeds

Heat the oil in a large sauté pan over medium heat. Add the garlic and ginger and sauté for 2 minutes. Add shrimp and sauté for 1 minute. Add slaw veggies, mirin, and tamari, stirring well to coat, and sauté 1–2 minutes until shrimp are just cooked through and veggies are hot and just wilted, but still crunchy. Remove mixture from heat, add sesame oil if using, and seeds, and toss to coat.

*Mirin is a Japanese sweet wine condiment available in Asian markets, natural food stores, or the international foods section of large grocery store chains.

Satisfying Bacon-Stuffed Sweet Potatoes

4 servings

4	medium sweet potatoes or garnet yams*
4	eggs
½	teaspoon sea salt
¼	teaspoon cracked black pepper
½	teaspoon minced rosemary (fresh or dried)
½	cup finely chopped cooked bacon or sausage
2	tablespoons finely chopped shallot

Preheat the oven to 400°F.

Thoroughly scrub and dry the sweet potatoes. Arrange the potatoes on a foil-lined baking sheet and cook for about an hour or until tender. Store them in the fridge to chill for later preparation or cool them slightly until you can handle the potatoes easily.

Set the oven to 350°F.

Using a sharp knife, cleanly slice off the very top of each baked potato and set aside. Carefully scoop out the flesh and set aside for another use (chilled cooked sweet potato is great in Basic Smoothies—see page 117 for recipe)—a melon baller works very well for this. Leave enough flesh inside the skin for the potato to hold its shape well. Arrange potatoes on a fresh foil-lined baking sheet.

In a small bowl lightly whisk together the eggs, salt, pepper, and rosemary. Add the meat and shallot and stir with a fork to thoroughly combine. Carefully spoon the egg filling into the cavity of each potato until it is nearly full. Bake for 20–30 minutes or until the centers are almost solid, but the mixture is still soft. Do not overbake. If your oven and potatoes are still hot from baking, the cooking time will be closer to 20 minutes.

*You may need a little more or less of the filling, depending on the size of the potatoes.

Savory Sirloin and Shiitake Salad

4 servings

For the Salad

1–1½	pounds sirloin steak (1 inch thick)
½	teaspoon each salt and cracked black pepper, or to taste, plus extra
2	tablespoons olive oil
8	ounces sliced shiitake mushrooms
2	shallots, thinly sliced
2	tablespoons slivered fresh basil (or 1 teaspoon dried)
6	cups chopped red leaf lettuce (or other hardy variety)

For the dressing

1	tablespoon sherry vinegar
1	teaspoon Dijon mustard
1	teaspoon lemon zest
	Pinches salt and fresh ground pepper, to taste
3	tablespoons olive oil

Preheat grill to medium high.

Season steak(s) to taste with salt and cracked black pepper. Lay the steak(s) on the grill and cook to desired doneness, about 4–5 minutes per side, depending on size, for medium rare.

While the steaks are cooking, heat oil in large sauté pan over medium heat. Add shiitake mushrooms and a couple of pinches of salt, and sauté 5 minutes. Add shallots and sauté for 2–4 minutes more or until the mushrooms and shallots are tender. Remove from heat and stir in basil.

While mushrooms are sautéing, in a small bowl, whisk together wine vinegar, mustard, lemon zest if using, and salt and pepper to taste, and whisk in oil to emulsify.

Slice the steak into thick strips. On a serving platter or individual plates, make a layer of lettuce, add the warm mushroom and shallot mixture, top with steak strips, and dress lightly to serve.

NOTE: To broil steaks instead of grilling, preheat broiler and lightly oil broiler pan. Set aside. Pat steak(s) dry, and season to taste with salt and cracked black pepper on both sides. Broil steak 3–4 inches from heating element for 4–5 minutes and turn. Broil for 4–5 minutes more for medium rare.

Simple Chicken Marsala

about 5 servings (set aside 1 serving for lunch)

2	tablespoons olive oil
2	pounds chicken tenders
	Sprinkles salt and freshly ground pepper
8	ounces sliced fresh mushrooms (any variety)
2	shallots, thinly sliced
¾	cup Marsala wine
¼	cup water
1	tablespoon minced fresh rosemary or ¾ teaspoon dried crumbled rosemary
1	teaspoon kudzu (or arrowroot or cornstarch) + 2 teaspoons water

Heat the oil in a large skillet or Dutch oven over medium heat. Add the chicken tenders and sprinkle lightly with salt and pepper. Cook for about 7 minutes or until cooked through but still juicy, turning frequently. Transfer to a dish and set aside.

Add the mushrooms to the pan and cook for 4–5 minutes until they release their juices. Add the shallots and cook for 2 minutes more. Add the wine, water, and rosemary. Reduce heat to low and cook for about 10 minutes. Increase heat slightly, if necessary to bring liquid to a simmer. Dissolve the kudzu into the 2 teaspoons of water and add to simmering liquid in the pan. Simmer for 1–2 minutes or until slightly thickened. Return the chicken to the pan and simmer for 3–5 minutes to warm the chicken and combine the flavors.

NOTE: Cooking wine is low-alcohol and 10 minutes of simmering will evaporate the alcohol content.

Sushi Salad

4 servings

For the Dressing

¼   cup sesame oil

¼   cup unseasoned rice vinegar

¼   cup chopped fresh ginger

1   tablespoon low-sodium, gluten-free tamari

2   teaspoons coconut nectar or few drops
     stevia, to taste

For the Salad

6   cups chopped romaine hearts (or baby
     spinach)

1   cucumber, chopped

1   large carrot, grated

4   green onions, sliced thinly

1   cup cooked brown rice, optional (room
     temperature)

1   pound cooked crabmeat pieces, claw or
     jumbo lump (or cooked salmon or shrimp)

1   large, ripe avocado, peeled, pitted and
     chopped

4   toasted nori sheets or ⅓-ounce prepared strips

To make the dressing, combine sesame oil, rice vinegar, ginger, tamari, and sweetener and blend with an immersion blender until smooth. (If you don't have an immersion blender, use a small regular blender or mince the ginger finely and whisk all ingredients together.)

In a large salad bowl, combine the lettuce, cucumber, carrot, green onion, cooked brown rice, crabmeat, and avocado. Pour the dressing over the salad and toss gently to combine. Shred the nori sheets or strips to top the salad just before serving.

Teriyaki Flank Steak

8 servings (set aside 4 servings for tomorrow's dinner)

¼   cup sesame oil

⅓   cup low-sodium, gluten-free tamari

3   tablespoons unseasoned rice wine vinegar (or rice vinegar)

    Juice of 1 lime

4   cloves garlic, minced

3   tablespoons grated ginger

2   tablespoons coconut nectar

1   teaspoon Dijon mustard

1   2-pound flank or skirt steak

Combine the marinade ingredients from the sesame oil through the Dijon mustard in a shallow glass storage container and whisk well to combine. Add the steak and turn several times to coat. Marinate in the refrigerator for 1 hour to overnight.

Grill the steak over medium high heat for 9–12 minutes, flipping once, for medium rare, or cook on the stovetop in a griddle pan over medium-high heat for 8–10 minutes, flipping once, or until it reaches desired doneness. To serve, cut the meat into thin slices, against the grain.

Tilapia over Wilted Baby Greens

4 servings

1	tablespoon coconut oil
2	large shallots, sliced
4	4-ounce skinless tilapia fillets*
	Sprinkles salt and freshly ground pepper, to taste
1	pint fresh blueberries (or other berries or chopped seasonal fruit)
6	ounces baby spinach, arugula, or a combination

Melt the coconut oil in a large skillet or Dutch oven over medium heat. Add the shallots and sauté for 2–3 minutes until soft. Remove shallots from skillet and set aside.

Reduce the heat to medium low and transfer the tilapia fillets to the pan. Sprinkle lightly with salt and pepper. Cook for about 4 minutes, gently flip, sprinkle lightly with salt and pepper, and cook on the remaining side for 4–5 minutes or until the fish flakes easily with a fork. Transfer the fillets to a platter and set aside in a warm place.

Add the blueberries, baby greens, and shallots to the pan and cover for 1 minute. Remove cover and stir gently, cooking for about 2 more minutes or until hot and greens are wilted. To serve, make 4 beds of the wilted greens and blueberries and top each bed with 1 tilapia fillet.

*Make one extra fillet for lunch tomorrow, if desired.

Snacks and Specialty Items

Almost-Instant Chocolate Protein Pudding

1 serving

1	scoop unsweetened chocolate protein powder (or vanilla)
1	tablespoon ground flaxseed
1	tablespoon dark cocoa powder
1	tablespoon almond butter
¼	cup unsweetened chocolate almond milk (or vanilla almond milk)
¼	teaspoon liquid vanilla stevia

Combine all ingredients in a small bowl and whisk until well combined and very smooth. Optional: add ⅓ cup of canned pumpkin puree (unsweetened) for a heartier snack.

Basic Bone Broth

3–4 quarts

For chicken stock

carcass of 1 or 2 chickens (including neck, any leftover skin, cartilage, and all bones)

For beef stock

4 to 6   meaty, marrow-filled beef bones (about 3 pounds)

For seafood stock

heads, tails, and bones from 4 small fish or 8 fish heads (or substitute shells from 1–2 pounds shrimp or lobster for 1–2 of the fish)

*Cold water

2   tablespoons apple cider or red wine vinegar

Place one set of bones (chicken, beef, or seafood) into a 6–7-quart slow cooker. Cover completely with cold water to about 2 inches from the top of the slow cooker insert.

Add the apple cider or red wine vinegar (to help the bones release their collagen).

Cook at least 8 hours to overnight on low.

The next morning, strain out all solids and discard.

Cool the stock in the refrigerator and skim off the top layer of congealed fat or foam. Use immediately or freeze in 2- and 4-cup portions in gallon-sized zip-closure freezer bags labeled with the date.

*For a more flavorful broth, you can add a couple carrots and celery stalks, preferably with the greens, and a whole sweet onion, unpeeled and quartered, to the slow cooker before adding the water, but it's not necessary.

Basic Green Salad

4 servings

For the Basic Balsamic Vinaigrette*

1   tablespoon high-quality balsamic vinegar

1   teaspoon Dijon mustard

1   clove garlic, minced, or 2 teaspoons minced shallot, optional

1   tablespoon fresh minced basil, optional

    Few pinches of salt and freshly ground pepper

3-4 tablespoons extra virgin olive oil

For the salad

4-6 lightly packed cups mixed greens (any lettuce, arugula, baby spinach, escarole, chicory, etc.)

2-3 cups chopped mixed salad veggies (mushrooms, shredded carrots, cucumber, red onion, radicchio, artichoke hearts, hearts of palm, Jerusalem artichoke, jicama, etc.)

1   cup chopped seasonal fruit (berries, melon, apple, pear, orange, etc.) optional

2-3 tablespoons nuts or seeds, optional

In a large salad bowl, whisk together all vinaigrette ingredients from vinegar through pepper to combine. Slowly add the olive oil while continuing to whisk until lightly emulsified. Add salad ingredients and toss well to lightly coat. Serve immediately.

*Making your own salad dressings is easy and inexpensive and the fresh flavor is far superior to anything you can find in a bottle. Vinegars keep virtually indefinitely, so when you see something that looks interesting buy it and add it to your collection.

To make the simplest vinaigrette, combine 1 part vinegar with about 3 parts oil in a glass or stainless steel bowl. Use more vinegar for a stronger flavor, less for a milder flavor. Add a few sprinkles of sea salt and freshly ground pepper and whisk to emulsify.

Oil and vinegar by their nature don't come together easily, so you can also use some emulsifiers to help. A little bit of mustard, raw honey, or fruit-sweetened jelly all work well as binders in vinaigrettes.

Basic Dairy-Free Pesto

about ⅔ cup

1	packed cup fresh basil (or ¾ cup cilantro)
1	loosely-packed cup baby or chopped spinach (or baby arugula, for a peppery bite)
¼	cup pine nuts, raw or lightly toasted (or walnuts, for a bitter note, or almonds)
2–3	teaspoons lemon juice, red wine vinegar, or balsamic vinegar, to taste
1–3	cloves garlic, crushed, to taste
¼	teaspoon salt, or to taste
⅛	teaspoon freshly ground pepper, or to taste
1	tablespoon rice miso or nutritional yeast, optional for a "cheesier" flavor
¼	cup high-quality olive oil

Combine the basil, spinach, pine nuts, lemon juice or vinegar, garlic, salt, pepper, and miso or nutritional yeast, if using, in a food processor and pulse several times to break up the greens. Scrape down the sides, add the olive oil and process to desired consistency. Taste and adjust seasonings, if necessary. Add more oil a teaspoon at a time for a thinner consistency.

NOTE: Pesto is very flexible and can be made with many different kinds of greens, nuts and oils. For some variety, try swapping out the basil for fresh cilantro and lime juice for the lemon. You can also use baby rocket arugula in place of the spinach for a peppery bite, or walnuts for pine nuts to lend a pleasant bitter flavor note.

Basic Sauerkraut

about 6 cups sauerkraut

1   large, fresh green cabbage, outermost
    leaves removed and set aside, cored and
    quartered (about 2½ lbs., cored)

2   tablespoons sea salt

2   teaspoons caraway seeds or 1 teaspoon
    cracked black pepper, optional

In the dishwasher,* sterilize a large mixing bowl (glass or enamel, avoid metal), 2 32-ounce Mason jars, tongs, a large spoon, and whatever you will be using to weigh the food down during the fermenting process. Wash your hands thoroughly before handling sterilized items and proceeding with recipe.

Slice the cabbage quarters finely, widthwise, to get thin strips, approximately ¼ inch wide by 2–3 inches long. You should end up with about 7 cups. (You can use the slicing attachment on your food processor to speed this process, but make sure the strips are no thicker than ¼ inch and your processor bowls and blades have been sterilized in the dishwasher.)

Combine half of the cabbage and 1 tablespoon of salt in the sterilized bowl and mix well. Massage and knead the cabbage until liquid begins to form. Squeeze as much liquid as possible out of the cabbage and add the second half of the cabbage and remaining tablespoon of salt. Continue to knead and squeeze the cabbage until you have a good pool of liquid.**

Mix in caraway seeds or black pepper, if using, and pack the cabbage and all the juices into the two sterilized Mason jars, using the tongs and spoon to help. The liquids should cover the cabbage completely by ½ inch.** Leave at least 2 inches of airspace between the top of the liquid and the top of the jars. Use one of the outer cabbage leaves to tuck the shredded cabbage down under the liquid line. It will help to weigh the shredded cabbage to keep everything submerged during fermentation.

To help keep the vegetables submerged, you can top the cabbage with a small sterile glass or glass dish and drop in a clean rock or tomato paste can to weigh it down. You can also fill a new (clean) sandwich-sized zip-closure bag ¾ full with distilled water or cooled brining water.** Tightly seal another bag around the first to prevent leakage (using brine ensures that if it does leak, it won't ruin your salt ratio). Using a "water bag" will also help to seal the jar without creating a pressure problem as the cabbage ferments. Repeat with the second jar.

Use plastic wrap to loosely cover the mouth of each jar, place them into a pan with edges (in case they overflow), and cover with a clean, heavy dish or hand towel.

Allow the jars to sit, undisturbed, in an area out of direct sunlight that ranges from 65–70°F (no warmer or your kraut may spoil) for 2 weeks, checking every couple of days to make sure the liquid levels are high enough. Top off with cool brining liquid if there isn't at least half an inch of liquid above the cabbage. If you notice any mold forming on the top of the liquid, remove it with a sterile spoon.

Using a set of sterile, non reactive tongs, remove a small amount of the cabbage from each jar to taste at ten days (it will be less tart) to see how you like it. If you want a stronger flavor, carefully replace all coverings and leave the cabbage for a full 2 weeks. Warmer climate temperatures generate faster fermentation, while cooler temperatures generate slower fermentation.

Once your sauerkraut reaches the desired strength, remove the plastic and any weights and cover the jars with their Mason lids. Store covered in the refrigerator to stop the fermenting process. The sauerkraut will last for 2–3 months refrigerated. Serve cold or at room temperature.

*Use the sterilize setting on your dishwasher to destroy any microbes on all the utensils you will be working with.

**If your cabbage is not particularly fresh, it may be difficult to get enough liquid by salting and massaging. In that case, boil 1½ cups of water on the stove for 20 seconds, remove from the heat, and stir in 1 teaspoon sea salt until dissolved. Cool this mixture to room temp and use it to top off the cabbage after it is packed into the jars.

Creamy Frozen Fruit

4 servings*

1	cup unsweetened vanilla almond or rice milk
1	cup low-fat coconut milk
1–2	scoops vanilla protein powder, optional
10	ounces frozen mango chunks
10	ounces frozen peaches
	Several drops stevia, to taste**
	Juice and zest of 1 small lime, optional
¼	teaspoon ground cardamom, optional

Place all ingredients from milk through cardamom, if using, into an industrial-strength blender (if you don't have a power blender, you may have to do this in smaller batches or a food processor to cream the frozen fruit). Blend until smooth but not liquefied. You should be able to scoop it with a spoon. Serve immediately.

*Cut recipe in half for a smaller amount, if desired.

**For sweeter, creamier ice, add a ripe frozen banana, broken into chunks.

Snack-Size Berry Smoothie

1 serving

1	cup chilled green tea, unsweetened light coconut milk, or unsweetened vanilla almond milk
½	cup frozen berries, any type
1	scoop unsweetened vegan protein powder (hemp, rice, or a combination—avoid soy)
1	tablespoon ground flaxseed or hemp seed
1–2	teaspoons greens or reds powder,* optional to taste
1–3	teaspoons coconut oil
	Few drops vanilla stevia, to taste, or 1 pitted date
	Few ice cubes

Combine all ingredients in an industrial strength blender, such as Vitamix, Ninja, or Nutribullet, and blend until smooth.

*Reds and greens powders are phytonutrient concentrates made from an assortment of fruits and vegetables. There are many different types and brands on the market. Check your natural food store for several options.

Tangy Lemon Oat Bars

8 bars

7	fresh pitted Medjool dates
½	cup dried apple rings
½	cup raw cashews
¼	cup whole-rolled, gluten-free oats
2	tablespoons hemp seeds (or 2 more tablespoons oats)
¾	teaspoon ground ginger
2	tablespoons fresh-squeezed lemon juice
1	teaspoon lemon zest

Place dates, apples, cashews, oats, hemp seeds, ginger, lemon juice, and lemon zest in a food processor and pulse a few times to break up the larger pieces. Then process for 1–2 minutes, scraping down the sides a couple of times. At first the mixture will break down into finer and finer crumbs, then it will finally pull back together into a single large clump that will roll around in the processor. When the ingredients are well incorporated into a "dough," transfer into a 5 x 7-inch Pyrex dish (3-cup size)* and press it into one even layer. Slice into 8 bars to serve (chill the dish for 1 hour for smoother slicing).

*If you don't have a small rectangular dish, wrap the dough in a large sheet of plastic wrap and roll to desired size with a rolling pin before slicing.

Creamy Vegan Dressing

about ½ cup dressing

⅓	cup unsalted macadamia nuts
¼	cup pine nuts
¼	cup water
	Juice of 2 lemons
1	large, fresh pitted date (soaked for 10 minutes in water if it isn't soft and fresh)
2–3	cloves garlic, crushed, to taste
¼	teaspoon each salt and freshly ground black pepper
2–3	drops liquid stevia, optional, to taste

Combine all ingredients in an industrial-strength blender and blend until smooth, scraping down the sides as necessary. Dressing should be thick and creamy, but if it's too thick to blend, add a little extra water or lemon juice, 1 tablespoon at a time. Taste and adjust seasonings if needed. Dressing will keep in the refrigerator for several days.

When Cravings Strike

When giving up familiar and even beloved foods, it's inevitable that you will find yourself craving them at some point, especially if you have to give up a food forever (e.g. anything that contains gluten, if you have celiac disease). The thing to remember when these cravings arise is that they are only feelings and that the feelings will eventually pass. The acute phase of most cravings only lasts about 10 minutes, and nearly all cravings will resolve on their own within an hour, if you don't give in to them. Here are a few calming techniques to help you wait them out:

Drink a big glass of water. Sometimes a food craving is really thirst in disguise. If you are craving something cold, like ice cream, it is nearly always a need for more water.

Distract your taste buds with a "surprise" flavor. Sometimes having a couple of mouthfuls of something with a strong taste that is very different from what you are craving will disrupt the craving and it will disappear. If you want something sweet, for example, have a few bites of something salty, like a strong pickle. If you are hankering for something salty, have something very sour, like sauerkraut or lemon instead.

If you are having persistent sugar cravings, sometimes it helps to increase your protein intake and/or decrease your intake of fruit or grains, especially rice and oatmeal for a while. People with very sensitive blood sugar tend to have fewer cravings and a more stable appetite if they eat more protein and fewer sweet carbs, even though fruits and grains are natural, whole foods.

If you're craving flour-based foods such as pasta, bread, crackers, or other baked goods, it can help to increase your serotonin levels naturally. Serotonin is your body's feel-good hormone and it also helps reduce carb cravings. Moderate regular exercise can increase natural serotonin production. Shoot for half an hour of exercise five days per week. Rhythmic motion like walking is especially beneficial.

Research tells us that many cravings for "pleasure foods" kick in when the reward region of our brains is tripped. These triggers can be either internal or external, like seeing a picture of fresh-baked bread, getting a birthday party invitation, feeling sad or overwhelmed, or driving by your favorite restaurant. Just thinking about a personal trigger can start the physiological cascade of food lust. To counteract that, consciously focus your mind on your specific goals for ending your gut discomfort and healing your digestive system. Enlisting your mind in this way activates your prefrontal cortex, both quieting the craving and kick-starting your mental resistance. The more specific you are about your goals, the stronger your ability will be to resist temptation. Write down exactly what you want for your health and well-being and exactly what you need to do to get there. Keep a copy of the list nearby and when cravings strike, read through everything you've written down or at least scan the list in your mind.

CHAPTER 10

Ending the Program

Coming off of the Gut Restoration Program offers a unique opportunity to identify true food sensitivities. The program acts like a big reset button for the gastrointestinal and immune systems. After spending several weeks eating a low-allergen diet, taking probiotics, improving digestive capacity, repairing the lining of the digestive tract, and de-stressing, you'll have a fresh start in which to assess your reactions to food and your current symptoms. By challenging foods in the following outlined process, you will know if you have a true sensitivity to a particular food or if your reaction to it was the result of a dysfunction of the digestive system from leaky gut, lack of digestive fire, a pathogenic infection, or stress.

Let Your Symptoms Guide You

After you have completed four consecutive weeks of the Gut Restoration Program, assess your symptoms. If they have improved by 50 percent or less, it is highly recommended to continue the program for an additional four weeks and reassess your symptoms after that time. If you have longstanding issues, complex medical problems, or exquisitely sensitive systems, you may need to be on the program for several more weeks. It is not a personal failure or a failure of the program if you need to stick with it for a while longer. Taking the weeks and months to invest in feeling good, after a long period of feeling unwell, is worth the commitment.

If your symptoms have improved by 50–75 percent or more, it's time to come off the program and monitor your symptoms (see all the following details). If you don't feel certain about your improvement, don't hesitate to stay on the program for two more weeks before completing the program. If your symptoms rebound after leaving the program, get back on board for another four weeks.

For those of you whose symptoms have improved by 75 percent or more, it is time to end the program.

How to Transition from the Program to Everyday Life

- Discontinue gut-repair nutrients. They can always be restarted, but the goal is to be on minimal supplements while maintaining low to no symptoms. Next, reduce the amount of probiotic you've been taking, from 100 billion CFUs to 20 billion CFUs. The lower dose of probiotics serves to manage your beneficial bacteria. Stay on this lowered dose for thirty to ninety days, and then taper off. If symptoms return, it can be restarted.

- Take a half dose of enzymes and acid for one week (if you've been taking them) and then discontinue use. Enzymes can then be taken as needed—when you're having a large meal, for example, of if you've eaten a troublesome food.

Upon completion of the program, you will have a unique opportunity to reintroduce foods that have been eliminated from your diet in a strategic way that will unmask any true sensitivities. Your body will let you know which foods it tolerates well and which ones it doesn't. After several weeks of gut restoration and immune-balancing techniques, you'll have a clean slate on which to experiment. The information that you will glean from this process is priceless.

Reintroducing Food, Step by Step

- Start with a single food item—wheat, for example. The food should be in a pure form without many additional ingredients, such as whole-wheat pasta, crackers, bread, or cream of wheat.

- For *one* day, have two to three servings of the food. Then, avoid it again for another three days. Delayed sensitivities can take up to 72 hours to manifest, and it is important to wait and see if symptoms develop.

- During the day in which you are challenging your system with a particular food, and in the three subsequent days, watch for symptoms. You might experience the return of old symptoms or perhaps the arrival of new ones. Be on the look out for gas, bloating, cramping, pain, diarrhea, constipation, mood swings, headaches, skin rashes and itchiness, fatigue, brain fog, and hives.

- If you have symptoms, it is an indication that you are likely sensitive to a particular food, in which case you should eliminate it from your diet for an additional four weeks, and then rechallenge yourself. If, after that period, the food creates symptoms again, consider avoiding the food completely. If the reintroduced food does not cause any symptoms after three days, that food can be rotated back into your diet. For the first two to three weeks after reintroduction, have the food no more than every three days. After that, eat it as desired.

- Repeat this process with the next food. Following this schedule, a new food item will be challenged every four days. There is no particular order to follow. Start with the foods you have missed the most.

The importance of reintroducing one food item at a time, every four days, cannot be stressed enough. You have spent a lot of time on this program, so it is worth it to take a bit more time to collect data on your unique sensitivities.

After challenging single items, try various food combinations, such as wheat and cheese, tomatoes and cheese, and so on. Many people can handle single food items easily but run into problems with food combinations.

Managing Relapse

After several months of feeling good you might begin to notice that symptoms are returning. Relapse typically occurs for one of two reasons. The most common reason for relapse is the reintroduction of foods that your body is inherently sensitive to. You may be able to handle small quantities of these foods, and as time goes by, you may consume more of them. Inevitably, with increased consumption, your system will once again cascade into inflammation, immune overstimulation, and damage to the small intestine. Once healed, the small intestine is not bulletproof and needs to be respected. Here's how to avoid relapse:

- Trim back consumption of suspicious foods. You are likely overconsuming just one or two items.
- Begin to take two capsules of enzymes with food.
- Continue with a maintenance dose of probiotics.
- Monitor symptoms for one to two weeks. If symptoms are not dissipating, double up on probiotics and start gut-repair nutrients for four weeks.

The second most common reason for relapse is antibiotic therapy. If you are prescribed an antibiotic and want to avoid relapse, take a probiotic with 50–100 billion CFUs alongside the antibiotic and stay on the probiotic for three times the length of the antibiotic course. For example, with a three-day course of antibiotics, take a high dose of probiotics for nine days. Take the probiotics while you are taking the antibiotics. They will not interfere with the efficacy of antibiotic treatment and will help reduce side effects. After nine days, monitor your symptoms carefully.

If symptoms continue to manifest, stay on the higher dose of probiotics. Add two capsules of enzymes with meals and gut-repair nutrients for two weeks.

Conditions

Navigating the torrent of health information found on the Internet and from health-care providers can be arduous and daunting at best. In Section 3, the Gut Restoration Program is outlined from start to finish, and serves as a guide to improve your symptoms. The next step is to introduce additional actions that can be taken in conjunction with the Gut Restoration Program to suit your particular needs. This section explores common and specific conditions related to your digestive system, along with targeted nutrition, supplements, and lifestyle interventions that can also help. Please note that you don't have to do anything in addition to the Gut Restoration Program in Section 3. It is complete unto itself and will greatly alleviate your digestive distress. This section is all about additional self-care options, should you choose to explore any of them.

By following the recommendations of the Gut Restoration Program, you will learn how to keep your symptoms under control—or even say good-bye to them for good.

CHAPTER 11

Gastroesophageal Reflux Disease (GERD)

Gastroesophageal reflux disease (GERD), acid reflux, and heartburn are terms that are used somewhat interchangeably to describe what happens when stomach acid backs up from the stomach into the lower esophagus.

The unpleasant feeling of reflux is all too common, with the vast majority of Americans experiencing reflux at some point in their lives. However, most reflux is transient and self-limiting, which means it will go away on its own.

Yet for 30 percent of Americans, reflux occurs on a weekly or more frequent basis. Although this common problem is considered part of the "normal" digestive experience—because it happens so often—experiencing reflux on a frequent basis is not normal and does not represent optimal digestive function, ever. In this chapter, you'll find out more about this condition and what you can do about it.

The Real Cause of Acid Reflux

Contrary to popular belief, reflux in adults is not caused by too much stomach acid. It is rather a case of acid in the wrong place. The lower esophageal sphincter (LES), a ring that separates the bottom of the esophagus from the stomach, sometimes gets lax and opens when it is not supposed to, allowing acid and occasionally food to move out of the stomach and into the esophagus. Ouch!

These are some of the most common causes of reflux:

- **Drugs.** Many types of drugs can make it more likely that you'll experience reflux or worsening symptoms of reflux. Steroids, birth control pills, aspirin, nonsteroidal anti-inflammatory drugs (NSAIDs) such as ibuprofen, aspirin, and naproxen, nitroglycerine (given for chest pain), progesterone, provera (prescription progesterone replacement), diazepam (also known as Valium, often prescribed for anxiety), and theophylline (a drug used for asthma and pulmonary disease) have heartburn as a side effect.

⊙ **Clothing.** Tight-fitting clothing and tight waistbands can worsen reflux. For those of you who have been looking for an excuse to toss out your skinny jeans, here it is. Bending over at the waist after eating, bending over frequently, late-night eating, eating large meals, and lying down after eating large meals also trigger reflux symptoms.

⊙ **Pregnancy.** Reflux is very common in pregnancy with the combination of increased pressure against the lower esophageal sphincter (LES) from the growing baby and the presence of high levels of progesterone, which relaxes the LES.

⊙ **Overweight and obesity.** People who are overweight or obese experience reflux at greater rates than their normal-weight counterparts. This is due at least in part to increased pressure on the LES from extra weight. Optimizing body composition can go a long way toward alleviating symptoms. Although the Gut Restoration Program is not a weight loss plan, many people report losing extra weight on the program.

⊙ **Hiatal hernia.** This type of hernia is present in about 20 percent of those with reflux. Your diaphragm has a little opening, called a hiatus, through which the esophagus passes as it connects to the stomach. When you have a hiatal hernia, part of your stomach bulges (herniates) through the hiatal opening. Some hiatal hernias are quite small and minor, some are large enough to necessitate surgery, and then there is everything in between. Hernias that aren't large enough for surgery will do quite well with the recommendations here.

⊙ **Stress.** Constant anxiety plays an enormous role in the development of GERD symptoms, and people with GERD often notice that symptoms are worse during times of high stress. Tight deadlines, arguments, and clashes with partners or bosses can make you reach for the roll of Tums in your pocket. Stress management is a cornerstone, not only for improving digestive complaints but also for increasing overall health and well-being.

⊙ **Foods.** Certain foods can also worsen reflux. Spicy foods, orange juice, tomatoes and tomato-based foods, coffee and other caffeinated drinks, deep-fried foods, onions and garlic, mint and mint-flavored products, and chocolate all have links to reflux. If you consume any of these foods on a regular basis and experience reflux, you might want to try removing or reducing them to see if your reflux improves.

◉ **Hypochlorhydria.** In some cases, reflux can even be caused by low stomach acid, a condition known as hypochlorhydria. The LES stays closed when you have enough acid in your stomach and can creep open when acid is low. Quite likely, this is the exact opposite of everything you have ever heard about reflux. Remember the special cells in the stomach that make stomach acid? As you get older, these special cells slow down and stomach-acid production begins to drop off. It requires a Herculean amount of energy for these special cells to make stomach acid. If you throw in that you may be eating foods you are sensitive to and not getting adequate nutrition because you are not absorbing nutrients from your food well, you are setting the stage for all of your cells to be tired—particularly the energy-hogging, acid-producing ones. This translates into reduced acid output by the stomach.

When your stomach isn't making enough acid, the pH increases. The pH of the stomach should be quite low—around 1–2—to help break down food, absorb vitamins and minerals, and keep infections at bay. In addition, low pH can create trouble for the LES. The LES struggles to stay tightly closed when levels of stomach acid are low. When those levels increase, the LES creeps open and allows whatever acid is in your stomach to splash up into the esophagus and create the symptoms of heartburn. Before you reach for your purple pill, read on . . .

The High Cost of Acid-Blocking Drugs

Consider this: Americans spend $3 billion on over-the-counter antacids such as Tums and Rolaids, over-the-counter acid blockers such as Prevacid and Tagamet, and a whopping $13 billion on prescription acid-blocking drugs. These drugs are good at reducing symptoms in the short term but do little to correct the underlying problem. In many cases, acid-blocking drugs actually exacerbate the underlying problem and create new issues.

When you head for your medicine cabinet and pop an acid-blocking medication such as Prevacid, you drive down your stomach-acid production even further.

Originally, acid-blocking drugs, including proton pump inhibitors (PPIs) such as Prevacid, Prilosec, Protonix, and H2 antagonists—Pepcid, Tagamet, and Zantac, for example—were originally approved by the FDA for short-term use. These drugs were never meant to be taken for more than six to nine months. Sadly, they are often taken for far longer than that—and some doctors even recommend taking them for life. Many of these drugs are now available over the counter, which means that people can take them indefinitely, without being monitored by a physician and perhaps without understanding the implications of such long-term use.

The knock-on effect of the chronic use of acid-blocking medications and low stomach acid spreads further than the potential for reflux. The most common side effects of these drugs are constipation or diarrhea, flatulence, bloating, nausea, and abdominal pain, but they have effects that are far more insidious, including the following:

- **Vitamin depletion.** Many nutrients depend on adequate stomach acid for absorption, and so the long-term use of acid-blocking drugs can set the stage for depletions. Vitamins B12 and B6, folate, calcium, iron, magnesium, zinc, and beta-carotene rely on stomach acid for absorption into the body. Anemia, fatigue, and osteopenia (thinning of the bones that leads to osteoporosis) are commonly seen with long-term proton pump inhibitor (PPI) use.

- **Poor digestion.** Pancreatic enzymes, your special helpers that break down proteins, fats, and carbohydrates, are activated by stomach acid and perform their best in the presence of acid. So, when you turn off stomach acid, you also turn off enzyme function and efficiency. Overall, this has the effect of greatly disrupting digestive capacity. When your food cannot be broken down into teeny, tiny particles for the small intestine to absorb, not only are you blunting absorptive ability—i.e., worsening cellular energy and function and thus digestive function—but you are also setting the stage for gas and bloating.

- **Dangerous bacterial overgrowth and infections.** Stomach acid helps protect you from pathogens that induce food poisoning, chronic infection, and other unsavory characters such as parasites. So when you reduce your stomach acid, you reduce your capacity to fight against the bad guys that you accidentally eat. Not only that, you create an environment that favors the overgrowth of bacteria when your stomach acid is reduced. The use of PPIs creates a twofold risk for *Clostridium difficile* infection (a rather unpleasant bug that gives severe colitis and diarrhea). Are you ready for more? When you overuse PPIs and your full arsenal of stomach acid isn't available, it's easy for bad guys to set up shop. Thus, bacterial overgrowth of the stomach and small intestine is a common complication of chronic PPI use. The only place bacteria belong is in the large intestine, so when they are found in other places, you are looking at trouble. Common signs that point to bacterial overgrowth of the stomach and small intestine are gas, bloating, belching, *H. pylori* infection, chronic yeast or bladder infections, and intolerance to fiber, carbohydrates, fructose-rich foods, and even probiotic supplementation.

- **Compromised resistance to superbugs.** In addition to encouraging *Clostridium difficile* infection, bacterial gastroenteritis, and bacterial overgrowth, acid-blocking drugs can increase your chance of being infected with an antibiotic-resistant superbug in a hospital setting and also increase the risk of community-acquired pneumonia by decreasing the activity of your bacteria-killing immune cells. In the elderly population, who are both at greater risk for community-acquired diseases and more likely to be on PPIs, these acid-blocking drugs can confer a worse prognosis.
- **Hip fracture.** Acid-blocking drugs can also increase the risk of hip fracture, which should come as no surprise, as these drugs deplete bone-building nutrients such as calcium, magnesium, and zinc.
- **Yeast infections.** Lastly, the environment that is created when stomach acid is reduced through overuse of acid-blocking drugs creates a friendly environment for yeast. Chronic urinary-tract infections, Candida overgrowth in the gut, and yeast infections are often seen with long-term use of acid blockers. Use them judiciously.

Additional Help for Gastroesophageal Reflux Disease (GERD)

The following are gentle interventions that you can implement in conjunction with the Gut Restoration Program (detailed in Section 3) to further target your specific concerns and conditions. When applicable, strategies for more targeted nutrition and supplementation are outlined, along with topics you may want to discuss with your doctor.

There is no right or wrong way to approach these additional recommendations. You may use all of them or just the ones that resonate with you. Some of them are simply good strategies to use for life (such as eating plenty of greens).

Additional food elimination. In addition to the items eliminated from your diet in conjunction with the Gut Restoration Program, it may be necessary for you to uncover which foods are triggering your symptoms. After a period of elimination and taking the time to heal your gastrointestinal tract, challenge any suspects one at a time to see who the culprit is (see page 172). At the outset, consider eliminating onion, garlic, cocoa, chocolate, oranges, and deep-fried foods.

Take a shot of apple cider vinegar before meals. One to two teaspoons of apple cider vinegar in some water before meals helps light digestive fire by stimulating the cells of the stomach to produce acid and increase enzyme output. If you don't like apple cider vinegar shots, have a small salad with a vinegar-based dressing before meals. Choose bitter greens for your salad because they also help to stimulate digestive fire—the body's ability to produce acid, enzymes, and bile to break down food.

Incorporate bitter greens into your daily diet. The use of bitter vegetables and herbs to spark digestive fire is a long-used natural approach to treatment of GERD. Eat plenty of dandelion greens, mustard greens, turnip greens, cress, and other bitter greens. These can be eaten raw, sautéed, or wilted into a warm salad. Supplemental bitter herbs, some of which taste very good, are readily available in health food stores. They are often found in tincture form—liquid in little glass bottles—and one full dropper before meals (about one teaspoon) will have an effect similar to apple cider vinegar. You can take the herbs "straight up" or wash them down with a few sips of water.

Consider cabbage juice. Yeah, that's right. Cabbage is a very rich source of glutamine, the preferential fuel for the cells that line the digestive tract—keeping them happy and productive—and helps soothe and heal the lining of the entire GI tract. An alternative to cabbage juice would be to make cabbage soup, then throw it into the blender, liquefy it, and use it as a base for soups or simply drink it several times per week.

Avoid mint and mint products. Mint causes the LES to dilate and is an often overlooked cause of symptom exacerbation. Try eliminating mint tea, mint lozenges, and mint-flavored gums, candies, toothpaste, and mouthwash. Don't worry, for sparkly clean breath, there are a variety of other options out there! Many toothpastes and mouthwash are made with cinnamon, neem, fennel, anise, xylitol, and/or baking soda.

Optimize body composition. Losing body fat will reduce the pressure on your LES, helping it to function better and stay closed. Try to eat as many leafy green veggies as possible, along with lean, clean protein, healthy fats, and low glycemic-index fruits such as berries, cherries, apples, pears, and pomegranate. Minimize tropical and citrus fruits.

Drink water! Bumping up your water consumption will have a plethora of beneficial effects, including reducing symptoms of GERD. Try to aim for at least 2.4 liters (80 ounces, or 5 pints) per day. This sounds like a lot, but once you get in the habit of drinking more water, it becomes effortless. Have 0.5–0.7 liters (16–24 ounces, or 2–3 cups) of water as soon as you wake up in the morning to help get you started.

Lifestyle Interventions

It's amazing what adopting a few new habits can do, not only for the way your tummy feels but also for mental clarity, emotional well-being, and overall health, as well. Some are easy "no-brainers" that you can do *right now*, while others may take time to cultivate and develop into habit.

- **Try a slow, restorative walk in the morning.** It will help balance the "fight or flight" branch of your nervous system with the "rest and digest" branch. In other words, a relaxing walk helps you to calm down and settle any stress. This in turn helps balance the enteric nervous system (ENS), the second brain of the body that lives in your gut and regulates digestive function—and which helps the lower esophageal sphincter (LES) remain closed so acid doesn't splash up into your esophagus and create heartburn symptoms. You can gain all of these benefits simply by talking a leisurely walk. Go out and smell the roses. And, if you have a canine friend, he or she would probably like to come along too.
- **Elevate the head of your bed by 6 inches.** Get a beam and place it under the head of your bed. This technique uses gravity as an aid to keep acid where it belongs. Once you have corrected the underlying reasons for your reflux, you can remove the beam.

⊚ **Consider getting visceral manipulation.** If you have a hiatal hernia—a condition that occurs when the stomach pushes through the diaphragm and traps acid in the esophagus—you can get a great deal of relief from various forms of massage and other types of tissue manipulation.

⊚ **Try Heel Drops.** To help adjust your hiatal hernia and get your stomach and esophagus back into the right position, do a heel drop. Here's how: In a standing position, take a big gulp of water and come up on your tiptoes. As you swallow, drop your heels to the ground. When you do this, the combination of the weight of the water plus gravity, as you drop down on your heels, will help set your hiatal hernia straight. Although this is a very simple technique, it gives great relief.

Supplements and Herbs

In addition to the supplements detailed in the Gut Restoration Program, there are several other good options. The following supplements should be used in conjunction with the Gut Restoration Program, however, if you choose to use them:

Replenish Stomach acid. Try supplemental hydrochloric acid (HCl)—but use it only if you do not have an ulcer. Reflux symptoms greatly improve with the use of supplemental acid, which seems to "wake up" the cells of the stomach and remind them to produce acid on their own. Contrary to what you may have been told before, it is possible for the body to regenerate, heal, and pick up normal function when given the right inputs. As a consequence, long-term supplementation (more than a few months) is typically not necessary. Dosing schedules can be found on page 88. Consider remaining on supplemental acid, if necessary, according to symptoms after you've completed the Gut Restoration Program (page 59).

Slippery elm. Slippery elm is a demulcent herb, which means it is soothing, slippery, and capable of coating surfaces. Slippery elm has a long history of use for GI disorders and is known to calm and soothe irritated tissues with a protective coating. Slippery elm is extremely safe and available as a powder, in capsules, and even in lozenges. You can add a teaspoon of slippery elm powder into smoothies and nut butters or make into a tea by adding 1 teaspoon of slippery elm bark to 0.47 liters (2 cups) of water, simmering, the mixture for 20 minutes, and then straining it. You can make a quicker version by adding 2–3 teaspoons of slippery elm powder to 0.47 liters (2 cups) of water and letting it simmer for 10 minutes. You can use stevia to sweeten the tea, but many find it quite nice all on its own.

Meadowsweet. Meadowsweet is another demulcent herb, and like slippery elm, it is very safe. In fact, you can consume several cups of the tea every day. To make the tea, add 1–2 teaspoons of the dried herb to 0.24 liters (1 cup) of water. Bring it to a boil, then take the water off the heat and let the herb steep for 10 minutes. Sweeten the tea as you like.

Ginger. When you are in the clutches of heartburn, a cup of ginger tea can help ease acute symptoms. Use ½–1 teaspoon of powdered ginger or 1–2 tablespoons of grated fresh ginger in a cup of water. Bring the water to a boil, take it off the heat, and steep the ginger for 10 minutes. Sweeten the tea as you like and sip it while it's hot. If you prefer, you can serve it over ice.

Deglycyrrhizinated licorice (DGL) wafers. Like meadowsweet and slippery elm, DGL is a demulcent herb that coats, calms, and soothes irritated tissue. Chewed after a meal, DGL helps form a protective barrier against acid. DGL wafers can be bought at most vitamin and health food stores.

Chamomile tea. Just like ginger tea, a cup of chamomile tea can help reduce acute, immediate symptoms of reflux. It also has relaxing and stress-relieving effects. Chamomile tea is readily available in most food stores.

Ask Your Doctor

There is no getting around it: sometimes you have to be your own health advocate. Although they are thoroughly trained, doctors are not perfect and sometimes they overlook or miss a thing or two. Here we suggest topics that you may want to talk about with your doctor regarding your symptoms and/or condition.

Rule out *H. pylori* infection. *Helicobacter pylori* is a common bacterial infection that can underpin reflux and gastritis and should be ruled out in cases in which you are having a hard time getting symptoms under control and/or have been on acid-blocking medications for more than six months. *H. pylori* infection can also predispose you to ulcers, which is an important reason why it should be ruled out. Of course, if it is present *H. pylori* should be treated and eradicated.

CHAPTER 12

Constipation

Constipation is not the most glamorous topic and perhaps not something you would discuss at a cocktail party, but it is certainly a relevant subject. More than 25 percent of Americans suffer from constipation—a condition that afflicts people of both genders and all ages. Women are twice as likely as men to be constipated, and it is more common for folks over the age of sixty-five to be constipated than it is for younger people, including children. However, constipation is on the rise among children, and it is a very common cause of gastrointestinal distress in that age group. (See page 271 for a complete discussion of constipation in kids.) Doctors write more than a million prescriptions for constipation every year, and people in the United States spend roughly $725 million annually on laxatives. That is a lot of laxatives! The good news is that there are many simple and effective things that you can do to alleviate this common condition. You won't even have to chat about it at dinner if you don't want to.

What Is Constipation Anyhow?

The definition of constipation often depends on whom you ask; even health providers can have different criteria to define constipation. It can also be quite subjective—some people feel constipated if they don't go to the bathroom daily, and others feel constipated if they don't go weekly. Generally speaking, if you meet at least two of the six criteria for constipation on this list, you can consider yourself constipated:

1. Fewer than three bowel movements per week
2. Hard stool 25 percent of the time
3. Feeling as if you are not "done" 25 percent of the time
4. Sensation of obstruction 25 percent of the time
5. Having to use manual maneuvers 25 percent of the time (This is a polite way to describe the use of hands or tools to remove stools.)
6. Hard stool without the use of laxatives

Why Is Constipation Such a Problem?

If you're wondering why one-quarter of the U.S. population is having such a hard time going to the bathroom, you don't need to look farther than lifestyle choices in the majority of cases. Refined and processed flour and dairy products are enough to stop up almost anyone, and unfortunately, these foods are the backbone of the standard American diet. Consuming foods that you unknowingly have sensitivities to can be quite problematic too. Throw in chronic stress and dehydration, and you have the perfect storm for, well, you know . . .

The Wrong Food

In addition to what you do put into your mouth, it is also worth considering what you don't put down the hatch. If you are eating large amounts of processed and packaged foods that are grain and dairy based, it means that these foods are displacing other foods from your diet that could be helping with bowel function. Before the agricultural revolution, humans ate a high-vegetable diet with adequate protein, healthy fats, and low-glycemic fruits. These foods are largely absent from most of our plates today. An illustration of this is magnesium, a mineral that is commonly found in green vegetables and nuts and that helps keep the bowel relaxed and moving well. Magnesium deficiency is a common contributor to constipation that is worsened when magnesium-dense foods are not consumed.

Not Enough Water

With all of the soda, frappuccinos, and juice drinks that Americans consume, there is less room for water. How many times have you heard someone say "I don't like the taste of water," or "I'm just not thirsty"? Hundreds of times, probably. If you are chronically dehydrated because you don't drink enough water and are consuming beverages that actually make you drier, gut motility will suffer.

Relaxation vs. Exercise

Regular physical movement helps keep the bowel regular—and yet, who can't relate to not finding the time to exercise because of long hours at work, trying to catch up on sleep, spending time with family or relaxing?

For many of us, *relaxing* means "hanging out on the couch surfing the channels or sitting and surfing the web." You may think these activities are relaxing, but in fact, they are far from it because they keep the brain overstimulated and unable to decompress. When you don't move, your bowels don't move either. Exercise is just as important as other forms of relaxation for bowel regularity.

Stress

Stress and living in our chaotic, fast-paced world can have a huge impact on bowel regularity. Your nervous system acts like a big seesaw, swinging between sympathetic "fight or flight" mode and parasympathetic "rest and digest" mode. If you are constantly in the stressed-out fight or flight mode, the sympathetic branch of the nervous system becomes dominant and bullies the rest and digest branch out of the way.

The result of this bullying is that the ability of the enteric nervous system (ENS), the so-called second brain that resides in your gut and controls its functions, to regulate peristalsis (the rhythmic, wavelike contractions that propel food down and out through the digestive tract) and normal bowel movements become impaired. Stress grinds us to a halt on multiple levels. Overbearing bosses, fights at home, too many deadlines, too many e-mails—and not enough time to do any of it (or even knowing where to start)—can all add up to make you feel so overwhelmed that you can't go to the bathroom.

Not Taking the Time to "Go"

Ignoring "nature's call" will also contribute to constipation. Not everyone is going to want to use the restroom at work, school, or while out shopping, and that is totally understandable, but when you get the urge, it's best to go. When you ignore your body's signals, eventually the body will stop sending signals and simply back up.

Medications

There is also a laundry list of medications and supplements that can slow us down. Opiates and antidepressants interfere with gut motility (the motion and activity of the gut), a depressing thought in itself. Calcium-channel blockers taken for high blood pressure and too many calcium supplements, iron supplements, aluminum-containing antacids, and laxatives also contribute to constipation.

Other Functional Issues

Chances are, if you are reading this book you may not have had great success with conventional ways of managing your gastrointestinal discomfort, or perhaps you are looking for alternatives. If this is the case, it is quite likely there is an underlying, as-yet-undiscovered issue with your gut that is contributing to your symptoms. Contenders might include bacterial dysbiosis, an imbalance between the good bacteria and the bad bacteria that live in your large intestine; small intestine bacterial overgrowth (SIBO), which occurs when bacteria set up shop in the small intestine where they shouldn't be; leaky gut, which contributes to inflammation, immune dysfunction, food sensitivities, and potentially, malabsorption of nutrients; dysregulation of the enteric nervous system (ENS), which slows down peristalsis (the transit of food through the GI tract); and nutrient insufficiencies, particularly magnesium and folate.

Associated Conditions

A number of other conditions are associated with constipation:

- **Hypothyroidism**, which occurs when the thyroid produces low levels of thyroid hormone, causing slower metabolism, cold intolerance, weight gain, muscle and joint pain, brain fog, dry skin, and thinning of hair and eyebrows
- **Hashimoto's thyroiditis**, in which thyroid function is lowered because the immune system is targeting the thyroid gland for destruction
- **Multiple sclerosis (MS)**
- **Diabetes**
- **Kidney disease**
- **Scleroderma**, in which the immune system targets the skin and certain organs, creating a body-wide buildup of scar tissue
- **Parkinson's disease**
- **Colon cancer**

Additional Help for Constipation

As you can see, the reasons for chronic constipation are many and can be multilayered. Thus, it is important to take a deeper look into contributing factors and consider making a few optional adjustments to your diet (including supplements) and exercise while you are on the Gut Restoration Program (see page 59). None of the following suggestions are required! They are simply options that you may enjoy and benefit from as you work through the program.

Dietary Interventions

Cut back on brown rice, apples, and bananas. If you are eating these foods daily (they can be constipating), you may want to consider eating them less frequently until symptoms improve, and then challenge them one by one to see if they slow you down.

Have a shot of apple cider vinegar. To help increase your digestive fire, consider having a splash of apple cider vinegar before meals or in salad dressing. Eat bitter greens several times weekly.

Incorporate fermented foods into your weekly nutrition. Foods such as sauerkraut and kombucha add beneficial probiotics and enzymes that can help get you moving.

Eat more watery veggies and fruits. It sounds like such a simple thing to do, but eating vegetables and fruits, such as cucumbers, pears, celery, lettuce and other green leafy veggies, spinach, zucchini, kiwis, blueberries, and strawberries will add to your overall water intake over days and weeks. Dehydration is a major cause of constipation, and it's nice to know that you don't have to drink all of your water—you can eat some of it too.

Make sure that you are eating healthy fats daily. Avocado, avocado oil, olives and olive oil, coconut, coconut products and oil, nuts, seeds and their butters, fatty fish, fish oil, cod liver oil, egg yolks, and fats from pasture-raised and grass-fed meats, are all options. Healthy fats help lubricate the GI tract and ensure easy passage of stool.

Drink at least eight 0.24-liter (8-ounce) glasses of water daily. Period. Start your day with a 0.47-liter (16-ounce) glass of water when you get up in the morning. This can really help stimulate the bowel.

Lifestyle Interventions

Create a bathroom routine. Each morning, set aside 10–20 minutes to sit quietly on the toilet without being interrupted, even if you do not have a bowel movement. You may feel quite silly sitting there or think it is a waste of time, but it will help retrain your gut and nervous system to relax and "let go."

Don't ignore the urge to go. Even if you are out in public! Yes, most of us would prefer to be in the privacy of our own home to poop. We totally get it, but don't squander the chance to go by holding it in. For those of you who really can't tolerate public restrooms, try listening to your iPod to distract yourself while you're there. It may sound like an odd solution, but it helps. Ignoring the urge to go will compound your constipation problem and keep you stuck.

Reduce stress. A major, often undiscussed cause of constipation is stress. Take a hard look at your stress levels and consider some management techniques such as these, for example: deep breathing; Tai Chi; contemplative walks; reframing situations (i.e., finding the silver lining in even the worst situation); changing perspective and thought patterns by using tools such as gratitude and giving people who "stress you out" the benefit of the doubt; finding the silver lining in even the worst situation; practicing mindfulness; being "in the moment," rather than stressing about the past or fretting unnecessarily about the future; and getting rid of toxic relationships. There are stacks and stacks of excellent books on the subject of self-realization and stress management by writers such as Byron Katie, Miguel Ruiz, Eckart Tolle, and Brene Brown, among others, that can change your life.

Regular exercise helps you go. In other words, if you move, your bowels will move. A mixture of weight training, sprints, burst-type activity, walking, and plyometrics can help improve constipation by helping to reset the nervous system, massaging the intestines, and firing up metabolism. If you are currently exercising and are experiencing constipation, it's time to switch up your flavor of exercise to stimulate things in a new and different way.

Get enough sleep. Sleep is a major reset button for our physiology and hormonal processes. During sleep, the rest and digest branch of the nervous system becomes active, helping your body heal and repair. During sleep, the stress hormones cortisol, epinephrine, and norepinephrine are reset for the day, helping to buffer your brain and body against any negative effects from excess stress. Stress hormones, as we have learned, can interfere with not only your ability to go to the bathroom but also your ability to be free of pesky gut troubles such as gas, bloating, spasm, and stomach pain. Leptin, a major gut hormone that acts as the fuel gauge for the body, signaling when you have had enough to eat and helping control appetite and satiety, is also rebooted while you sleep, giving you a fresh slate to start the day. These are just some of the factors why sleep is a major player in the regulation of the digestive system.

Supplements and Herbs

Slowly increase fiber intake. The golden rule with fiber supplementation is "Start low and go slow." Eating too much fiber too fast can actually worsen constipation, the exact opposite of what you want to do. Acacia-based products are fabulous for constipation. Use either product once or twice daily, starting with ½ teaspoon in water, and increase the amount by ¼–½ teaspoon every five to seven days until you are using 2 tablespoons once to twice daily. It is very important to increase your water intake when you take supplemental fiber. You can't add extra fiber to a dry system and expect it to help move the bowels. Too much fiber with too little water will worsen constipation, so drink up!

Take magnesium daily. Magnesium, which most people don't get nearly enough of in their daily diet, helps the musculature and nervous system of the bowel relax; it aids peristalsis and helps improve bowel regularity. In addition, magnesium performs more than 400 other metabolic services for the body, every day. Foods that are rich in magnesium include cocoa powder, dark chocolate, seeds of all kinds, tree nuts and butters (especially Brazil nuts and almonds), and caviar. Incorporate these foods into your daily diet, and if you want to try a magnesium supplement, consider magnesium glycinate, which is well absorbed and gentle. Start with 200 milligrams before bedtime and work up to 400 milligrams, over several days or weeks. High doses of magnesium (typically more than 700 to 800 milligrams) can have a laxative effect.

Try vitamin C to shake things up. Did you know that vitamin C can be used as a laxative and a stool softener? It performs a multitude of other functions as well, including helping the body to build collagen and soft tissue and boost immune function. When you use vitamin C as a digestive aid, it's all about finding your upper tolerance level—the amount of vitamin C you have to take to get things going. To do this, start with 500 milligrams twice daily, and double this amount every one to two days. Once you find your vitamin C tolerance level, you may use it on an as-needed basis. Unlike commercial laxatives and even some herbal laxatives, this method does not create dependency. Vitamin C comes in a wide range of forms, from chewable tablets to powders to capsules. You can choose the form you prefer. Note that many vitamin C products have a lot of sugar in them, so you will want to steer clear of those. Capsules may be your best bet in that regard, and they are often conveniently packaged with 500 milligrams of vitamin C per capsule.

Consider taking more digestive enzymes with meals. Taking more enzymes—not acid—with meals can help stimulate bowel function. In people with chronic constipation, taking an extra capsule of plant digestive enzymes in addition to the recommended two capsules with meals will help to get things moving along. Full details on how to choose a digestive enzyme are outlined on page 86.

Herbal laxatives are acceptable, but don't use them every day. Using a product such as Smooth Move tea or Swiss Natural Herbal Laxative at dinner or before bed and following the other lifestyle tips in this section will help stimulate a bowel movement. However, laxatives—even herbal ones—should be used only as a support measure and not every day. In order not to create dependency, don't use Smooth Move or Swiss Natural Herbal Laxative for more than seven days in a row, initially, or more than two to three times weekly thereafter.

Serotonin is commonly thought of as a neurotransmitter. This means it appears to be exclusively made and utilized in the brain, but your digestive tract makes about 90 percent of your body's serotonin! In fact, your gut also has more serotonin receptors than your brain, which means it is especially sensitive to serotonin, whose job is to help regulate peristalsis and gut motility. In other words, serotonin helps food move through the digestive tract and helps you have regular bowel movements. Research suggests that people who have chronic constipation or the constipated type of irritable bowel syndrome (IBS) have suboptimal levels of serotonin. Consequently, the use of serotonin building blocks and receptor-sensitizing agents can help with constipation and restart peristalsis—it is like a set of jumper cables for the enteric nervous system (ENS)—and include the B vitamins, magnesium (there's magnesium again!), and 5-HTP 5-hydroxytryptofan (5-HTP), a building block of serotonin. In addition, SAMe, L-theanine (a medication used for anxiety and depression), and St. John's wort sensitize the body to serotonin and help it become more receptive to serotonin's message: "Get those bowels moving." These compounds are often found together in serotonin-support formulas. If you are on an antidepression medication, however, it is important to talk to your doctor about the use of 5-HTP because you may not tolerate it well when combined with antidepression medication.

Ask Your Doctor

The following is a list of topics to discuss with your doctor—conditions that you want to rule out or medications that have constipation as a side effect, in which case you may want to explore alternatives.

Rule out bacterial dysbiosis, infection with Candida, and parasites. I know that thinking about these things can make one squeamish, but unfortunately, they can all create and compound constipation and are often overlooked causes. A comprehensive digestive stool analysis (CDSA) will definitively rule in or rule out these factors. If you do have one of these pathogens on board, see page 215 for information about how to deal with it.

Rule out small intestinal bacterial overgrowth (SIBO). This is done with a breath test that your doctor can order for you. SIBO is a significant cause of chronic constipation and should be eradicated if you have it. Other symptoms that you may have SIBO are bloating; belching; and intolerance to fiber, carbohydrates, and probiotic supplements. If you do indeed have SIBO, see page 209 for the protocol to eradicate it. See page 303 for information on breath testing and labs that offer it (if your doctor is unsure or unwilling to give you the test).

Antacid medications. If you have used these for a long time, it is time to consider getting off of them! Constipation is a notorious side effect of long-term antacid use. (See pages 180–184 for tips.)

Take a hard look at your medications. Research the side effects of any medications you may be taking. Drugs.com is a great website to use for researching the side effects of all drugs on the market. For a list of commonly prescribed drugs that cause constipation, see the introduction to this chapter on page 176. If you are taking any of these medications, discuss alternative drugs with your doctor. Advocate for yourself. It is your body, and you are the one that has to live inside of it.

Get your thyroid checked. Thyroid dysfunction can greatly impact bowel function. Other than constipation, symptoms of thyroid dysfunction include cold intolerance; muscle and joint pain; dry skin and hair; and thinning eyebrows. The typical screening for thyroid function is a thyroid stimulating hormone (TSH) test, but it can miss a good chunk of thyroid dysfunction. Ask for free and total T3 and T4 (the active and inactive forms of thyroid hormones), rT3 (reverse T3) and autoantibodies anti-TPO (anti-thyroid peroxidase) and anti-TG (thyroglobulin). You want to get as much information on the state of your thyroid as you can, rather than a simple screening test.

CHAPTER 13

Inflammatory Bowel Disease (IBD)

It is estimated that up to 2 million Americans have inflammatory bowel disease (IBD), an umbrella term that covers a few individual and unique diseases: Crohn's, ulcerative colitis, and microscopic colitis (lymphocytic and collagenous)—all three of which have a slightly different presentation and symptoms, and each affects a certain portion of the gastrointestinal (GI) tract somewhat more than the others. The overarching theme of IBD is inflammation, and it is present in all of these conditions to the point of tissue destruction.

IBD lends itself extremely well to the Gut Restoration Program (see page 59) because the program strikes at several underlying causes of IBD—dysbiosis (the imbalance of good, beneficial bacteria and harmful, pathogenic bacteria), food sensitivities, leaky gut (when the lining of the small intestine loses its integrity, creating an abnormal immune response), inflammation, the propensity for food sensitivities and autoimmunity to crop up, a host of body-wide symptoms, and an overly strong and frankly dysfunctional immune response. IBD is a chronic disease, which means that in many cases it cannot be completely eradicated, but once you have addressed the underpinning causes and take measures to control symptoms, it is entirely possible to heal the intestine, get normal results from colonoscopy, and feel much, much better.

Causes and Symptoms of Inflammatory Bowel Disease (IBD)

IBD is thought to have an autoimmune component, although the mechanism that explains how it works is still being researched. Essentially, IBD boils down to an abnormal immune attack against normal food and bacterial compounds that are found in the gut: Your body reacts strongly against certain foods you are eating—usually grain- or dairy-based foods—and acts even against the friendly, beneficial bacteria that live in the large intestine. This reaction, or attack, begins to degrade the protective lining of the gastrointestinal tract, causing ulceration or even open wounds. Additionally, leaky gut, a loss of integrity and subsequent hyperpermeability in the lining of the small intestine, is very common in those with IBD. Sadly, leaky gut further spurs an abnormal inflammatory response, which keeps the whole cycle going. As such, a major consequence of IBD—besides open wounds in your intestines—is malabsorption of nutrients and subsequent malnutrition and nutrient insufficiencies.

Symptoms of IBD can range from mild to debilitating and sometimes disappear for months and even years, much to the mystification of doctors and researchers alike. Abdominal pain and cramping are common, as well as bloody diarrhea, frequent bowel movements and the sensation that you may have an accident if you don't find a bathroom RIGHT NOW, rectal bleeding, and tenderness of the belly. Constipation can also be a part of the IBD picture, along with broad, body-wide symptoms such as fever, weight loss, and inability to gain weight. In children, an inability to gain weight—or a lower-than-expected rate of weight gain and growth—is referred to as "failure to thrive."

Scientists are debating whether IBD is triggered by factors such as these:

- Infection
- Loss of tolerization to friendly bacteria
- Inflammation of the blood vessels in the gut
- An overblown reaction to something the immune system "sees" in the gut, such as tissue, food, or bacteria

As researchers go back and forth debating which theories hold water and which don't, you can begin to tackle some of the underpinnings of IBD by completing the Gut Restoration Program and utilizing the additional tips found at the end of this chapter.

IBD, Genetics, and Birth Control

IBD can run in families, and it is more common in women who take birth control pills. If you are taking oral contraceptives and someone in your family has IBD, you may want to consider another form of birth control. It appears that using oral contraceptives can induce IBD in those who are genetically prone to it.

Crohn's Disease

Diagnosis of Crohn's disease is on the rise in Western as well as developing countries that have adopted a diet that is high in refined carbohydrates. Rates of diagnosis are thought to be five times higher than that for ulcerative colitis. Crohn's diagnosis is strongly correlated to a higher-than-normal intake of refined carbohydrates and sugar.

The major symptoms of Crohn's disease are diarrhea, weight loss, and spasmodic abdominal pain. Pain can often be present near the ileum or ileocecal valve, near the right hip, aiding in diagnosis. Periods of constipation are common with Crohn's. Fever, canker sores, and clubbed fingernails can also be present. The disease can affect any part of the GI tract, yet it commonly affects the ileum, the final section of the small intestine. If imaging is done on the GI tract, "skip lesions" are often seen, which helps differentiate Crohn's from ulcerative colitis (UC). Skip lesions occur when inflammation penetrates the wall of the intestine, sometimes giving the appearance of a quilt, where patches of healthy, normal tissue are interspersed with patches of irritated, red, inflamed tissue. In Crohn's, inflammation penetrates deeper into the wall of the intestine than it does in ulcerative colitis.

Ulcerative Colitis (UC)

Ulcerative colitis (UC) is not as common as Crohn's disease and seems to be driven by an autoimmune response. Some studies suggest that in many patients with UC, the immune system attacks the large intestine by making antibodies against the cells of the large intestine. Symptoms are quite similar to Crohn's, although bloody diarrhea is more frequently seen in UC.

A differentiating factor between UC and Crohn's is that UC much more commonly affects the colon and rectum, as opposed to Crohn's, which often affects the last portion of the small intestine. In UC, the entire lining of the large intestine can be characterized by a pattern known as lead pipe, because, when it is imaged, there is so much uniform inflammation in the large intestine that it actually looks like a lead pipe, in contrast to the characteristic skip lesions in Crohn's, in which inflamed tissue "skips around" healthy tissue.

Lymphocytic and Collagenous Colitis

These types of colitis are known collectively as microscopic colitis and are relatively new kids on the block. Symptoms are similar to both Crohn's and UC: diarrhea, cramps, abdominal pain, fever, joint pain, and weight loss; yet when you take a look at the intestines with a colonoscopy, all of the tissue looks healthy—there is no obvious inflammation such as the kind that is seen in Crohn's and UC. However, if you examine a biopsy of tissue, taken from the intestines, under a microscope, you will see a greater-than-normal number of lymphocytes, a type of white blood cell (in lymphocytic colitis), or a thickening of the collagen layer—connective tissue under the lining of the intestine—with inflammatory molecules (in collagenous colitis). In either case, there are abnormal changes to the intestine on a microscopic level, rather than something that can be seen with the naked eye.

With lymphocytic colitis, quite often there is a single triggering incident such as an illness, virus, bacterial infection, or even a major stressor, such as unexpected death or trauma, a divorce, or a car accident.

IBD and the Role of Dysbiosis

As we know, the gut is the seat of the immune system, housing 75 percent of our immune cells. We also know that our beneficial gut flora—microbiota—not only exert enormous influence over our immune system but have immune function themselves.

These facts have spurred researchers to look carefully at the relationship between IBD and the microbiota. What they have uncovered is an almost universal dysbiotic situation—an imbalance of good guys (beneficial bacteria) to bad guys (potentially harmful, pathogenic organisms) in people who have IBD. Dysbiosis, in turn, affects immune function, potentially creating an opening for autoimmunity and dysfunctional immune responses to set up shop. Under these circumstances, the immune system begins to attack normal, healthy flora and even food particles.

In the Gut Restoration Program (see page 59), a central approach to IBD management is the supplementation of beneficial bacteria. Emphasizing the colonization of *Lactobacillus* and *Bifidobacterium* strains of bacteria, and inhibiting the growth of *Clostridia*, *Bacteroides*, and *E. coli* bacteria is a common tactic utilized by savvy integrative health providers to manage the symptoms of IBD. Studies have shown that the benefits of using probiotics are considerable, and probiotics have been shown to induce remission and increase the amount of time spent in remission for people who have Crohn's, UC, and microscopic colitis.

When there is dysbiosis—an imbalance between beneficial bacteria and potentially harmful organisms—in the large intestine, levels of a compound called butyrate decline. Butyrate is one of many short-chain fatty acids made by our beneficial bacteria as they ferment and digest fibers from the food we've eaten. Butyrate is like an energy drink for the cells that line the GI tract. When butyrate is low, the cells become slow and do not replace themselves as readily as they should. As a result, they stay locked in the cycle of inflammation, which is the exact opposite of what you want.

IBD and Leaky Gut

The immune system is abnormally fired up in people who have IBD, as it releases inflammatory compounds and makes antibodies against food, normal flora, and even the cells that line the GI tract.

In response to these inflammatory molecules, the cells that line the small intestine "break formation." Remember how they are supposed to stand tightly together, shoulder to shoulder, like a row of soldiers? Well, inflammatory compounds cause this tightness to weaken, and the desmosomes, which we learned about in Chapter 3 (see page 26), to become unbuttoned. This allows more immune cells into the area as the lining is breached—a smart evolutionary tactic, right? If you had a bad guy in your gut that the immune system had to kill, you would want fast and easy access to immune cells to get there and kick some butt. That's why desmosomes can be unbuttoned in the presence of inflammatory immune molecules. However, inherent in this evolutionary stroke of genius lies a weakness. In chronic inflammation, such as IBD, those gaps never close, the desmosomes don't re-button, and thus leaky gut manifests.

Along with leaky gut (increased intestinal permeability) and the accelerated antibody production against anything and everything the immune system happens to meet, in IBD the building blocks of the gut wall—the brick and mortar that helps keep it together—are compromised. Collagen-building compounds called GAGs (glucosaminoglycans) are readily and rapidly degraded, compromising the gut even further and causing the intestine to feel as if it is on fire.

Additional Help for IBD

Although the mechanisms for the development of IBD are multifactorial and quite likely highly specific to the individual, there are a number of things that you can begin to incorporate in your day-to-day life right now that will help reduce inflammation in the gut, better manage symptoms, and even strike at the reasons why IBD showed up in the first place.

Dietary Interventions

Eat warm, cooked foods. Do this especially during a flare but continue eating them until you have had several months of stability. Minimize raw foods and cold foods. Fruits can be baked or turned into a compote, salads can be wilted and turned into warm salads, and raw veggies cooked in soups and stews. Warm, cooked foods are easier to digest and easier on the intestine. The fiber in veggies and fruits, when cooked, is easier to break down and assimilate.

Minimize histamine-containing foods. Histamine is the compound that is released when you have an allergic response. A survey of the members of the National Foundation of Ileitis and Colitis found that up to 70 percent of people who have IBD also reported allergy-related symptoms. So people who have IBD may find it is worthwhile to do a four-week trial elimination of histamine-containing and histamine-liberating foods to see if this reduces symptoms and/or quells flares. Yogurt, kefir, cultured cottage cheese, sauerkraut, kimchi, kombucha, wine, beer, and hard cheese contain high levels of histamine. Ironically, these fermented foods are often recommended for gut healing! Additionally, cured meats, yeast-containing foods, and mackerel pack a powerful histamine punch.

Other foods, including the citrus family (lemons, limes, grapefruit, tangerines, tangelos, etc.) and spinach liberate and raise histamine levels when we eat them, and potentially trigger IBD symptoms.

Consider a trial elimination of yeast-containing foods. A study demonstrated that a high percentage of people with Crohn's disease have antibodies to *Saccharomyces cerevisiae*, otherwise known as baker's or brewer's yeast. This is a different animal from *Saccharomyces boulardii*, yeast that is used to actually target and kill pathogenic yeast and bacterial infections and is not correlated with Crohn's or other types of IBD. Hang on, you may be thinking—yeast that kills yeast? Yes, that's right. It's just like using a cat to hunt mice. Cats and mice are both mammals, but they are very different species. It's the same with yeast. If you remove foods from your diet that contain baker's and brewer's yeast, you are giving your immune system one less thing to contend with.

Use gelatin. Plain, Knox gelatin is a rich source of glutamine and other collagen-building blocks that help build a strong gut lining with good integrity. Gelatin also has a demulcent, slippery quality that is soothing to irritated gut mucosa. Make gelatin with herbal or berry teas instead of water, add it to smoothies or cocoa drinks, or use it in soups and stews to support the health of your gut and reduce inflammation and its symptoms.

Lifestyle Interventions

Avoid certain surfactants. These are used in soap, shampoo, conditioner, body wash, laundry detergent, dish soap, etc. Unfortunately, a wide variety of personal and household items contain dextran sodium sulfate (DSS), which is commonly used to induce colitis in mice and is known to irritate the intestine, and another surfactant, sodium lauryl sulfate (SLS). If any of the products you use contain DSS or SLS, swap them out for more natural brands that can easily be found, even in mainstream grocery stores. If you have IBD, using products with DSS or SLS is like rubbing your intestines with sandpaper.

Avoid thickeners such as carrageenan, and minimize the use of gums. Carrageenan is a thickening agent and conditioner that manufacturers add to many milk alternatives, helping to improve the body and texture of these products. Although carrageenan is made from algae, a seemingly innocuous compound, it has a shadow side because it can worsen colitis and prevent the lining of the intestine from healing. Other thickeners, such as guar gum and xanthium gum, are found in many gluten-free, processed, and packaged foods and can also cause GI irritation. The use of carrageenan and other thickeners is often the hidden cause of colitis or the hidden reason why symptoms aren't calming down. Read those labels carefully.

Supplements and Herbs

Consider taking probiotics every day. Even after you complete the Gut Restoration Program, probiotics are a good addition to your diet. One of the main facets of IBD is a significantly altered gut flora, and research is unsure if it is a trigger of, or a result from, the inflammatory process. To be on the safe side, it is recommended to take probiotics for the long term and certainly if you are on antibiotic therapy. If you have IBD, you may not tolerate large doses of probiotics very well, so go slowly and look for a product that works for you. For tips on choosing a probiotic, see page 84.

Take a high-quality multivitamin/multi-mineral supplement. This will help address nutritional insufficiencies and fill in the gaps that are not provided by diet alone.

Consider an antioxidant complex. Inflammation is the main driver of IBD and generates damaging free radicals that can injure DNA and cell membranes in a process called oxidative damage. If you can picture a metal bucket rusting outside in the rain, it is a good example of oxidative damage. Antioxidants help reduce this damage. A wide variety of antioxidants and antioxidant blends are available on the market. Look for a product that has 400 IU mixed tocopherols and tocotrienols (vitamin E), 200 micrograms selenium, 500 milligrams vitamin C, and 10,000 IU carotenoids to help stave off inflammation.

Consider the use of zinc. It helps particularly during a flare or bout of diarrhea. Taking 5 milligrams of zinc two to three times daily can help slow the bowel and blunt a flare. Zinc supplementation improves the function of the gut lining, and research shows it is especially efficacious in Crohn's disease.

Make curcumin a part of your everyday diet. Curcumin is the active part of turmeric, the bright orange spice found in curry and Indian cuisine. If you did a Google search for "curcumin and IBD" you would be overwhelmed by a multitude of studies, products, and blogs that tout the benefits of using turmeric. The praise is well deserved and solidly backed by research. Turmeric blocks all of the inflammatory mediators that drive the inflammatory response in IBD and has been shown to actually prevent the induction of colitis in mice. Turmeric itself is not well absorbed into the blood and remains in the GI tract instead, where it coats the inflamed intestines and acts as a balm. This is why it is a great idea to eat turmeric every day, particularly if you have IBD. It is totally acceptable, however, to take a supplemental capsule (1–2 grams, twice daily) if you can't or don't want to eat turmeric quite so often.

Curcumin, the active agent in turmeric, helps to reduce not just the inflammation from IBD but also the damage that the inflammatory process has already wreaked on your body. Curcumin is often sold in supplemental form as a capsule. It is worth noting that there are two main preparations of curcumin supplements, Meriva and BCM-95, which are particularly effective because they are bound to a phospholipid and are thus readily absorbed into the bloodstream and into your body. These supplemental forms excel at dealing with the systemic, body-wide issues that are a consequence of IBD. The bottom line is that taking both a supplemental form of curcumin and eating the spice turmeric daily will give you all the benefits of this powerful herb.

Curcumin has a variety of other beneficial side effects. When it goes head to head with conventional NSAIDs such as ibuprofen for musculoskeletal pain, curcumin wins every time. It is also fantastic for brain health, because it increases a molecule called brain-derived neurotrophic factor (BDNF). BDNF helps baby neurons form and make connections with other neurons, and it prevents neurons from dying prematurely. Curcumin also stimulates the NRF-2 pathway in the brain, which helps increase the brain's production of glutathione, a very powerful antioxidant. Much study is underway for the role of curcumin in cancer prevention and treatment. A typical dosing schedule for curcumin is 1 gram twice daily. Curcumin is safe at high doses. Good curry powders contain a high percentage of turmeric. Try the curried chicken salad suggestion in Week 1 for a quick meal (see page 107).

Dairy-Free Turmeric Milk

Turmeric is a common spice in Indian cuisine. In India, turmeric milk is often taken as a soothing remedy for joint pain or a sore throat. To make a dairy-free version, heat 1 cup of unsweetened coconut milk over medium heat and stir in 1 tablespoon of grated fresh turmeric root (or ½ teaspoon ground turmeric), 1–2 tablespoons of grated fresh ginger root to taste, 4 cardamom seeds, and 3 black peppercorns. Cook the mixture for about 5 minutes and then remove it from the heat. Cover and let it cool for about 10 minutes. Strain out the spices, sweeten the milk with a few drops of vanilla stevia, and serve it warm.

Increase omega-3 fatty acid intake. Specifically, bump up your intake of EPA and DHA in cold-water fish such as salmon, mackerel, herring, halibut, sardines, and tuna, all of which are excellent sources of omega-3 fatty acids and should be consumed several times weekly. However, if you have IBD and need a little extra help, it would be beneficial to take supplemental omega-3 fatty acids in the form of fish oil, krill oil, cod liver oil, or fermented cod liver oil. Taking 3–4 grams of combined EPA and DHA daily can reduce yearly remission rates of IBD by 50 percent. This dose can also significantly reduce daily symptoms.

Give bromelain a try. Bromelain is an enzyme that is found in the stems of pineapple and has been shown to reduce inflammation in people who have IBD. It is important to note that if you are allergic to pineapple you shouldn't take bromelain. For those of you who tolerate bromelain well, it has many other beneficial effects, including boosting the health of the respiratory system and calming an overstimulated, fired-up immune system. Take 2,000–3,000 milligrams per day. Bromelain is very safe, even in high doses.

Consider IgA supplementation. IgA is a non-inflammatory immune molecule that is one of the first lines of defense of the immune system. When we breathe in a virus, IgA attaches itself to it, almost like a Post-it note, signaling to the rest of the immune system: "Hey, guys, I've got something over here." IgA is found on all mucous membranes: in the mouth, throat, gastrointestinal tract, and genitourinary tract. In your gut, IgA helps keep the immune system calm and nonreactive to the food you eat and the beneficial flora that live in it. Though the data are mixed, it is thought that people with IBD have lower amounts of IgA, which contribute to the overstimulation of the immune system. Taking supplemental IgA—in the form of bovine colostrum —can help calm immune response and make the immune system friendly again to our microbiota and the food we eat. Tristan Biesecker of Biesecker Laboratories and Biesecker's line of products for Crohn's disease also advocates the use of raw milk to boost levels of IgA, unless, of course, you are sensitive to dairy products.

Try phosphatidylcholine (PC). There is a mucous layer in the large intestine (very much like the one found in the stomach) that plays a part in protecting the intestine from inflammation, abnormal immune response, and invasion by bad bacteria. Goblet cells secrete this protective layer, which is almost 90 percent phosphatidylcholine (PC). In IBD, there can be a deficit of goblet cells, which means the protective mucous layer can be reduced, as well. Supplementation of 2–4 grams daily of PC can help replenish lost amounts and spruce up the protective mucosal layer. PC is also great for brain and liver health and makes it easier for nerves to communicate with each other more efficiently.

Consider using aloe vera and other demulcent herbs. *Demulcent* means "soothing." Demulcent herbs work by creating a soothing barrier on irritated tissues that helps calm and soothe immune response and reduce inflammation. Many of them can also be used to rebuild the gastrointestinal lining. There have been multiple studies on these herbs. For example, a study of people drinking 100 milliliters of aloe vera juice twice daily for one month found it helped to heal the lining of the gut, decrease symptom frequency, and put 30 percent of participants into remission. Note that aloe vera juice can also be used as a laxative, so in this case—more is not better. Experiment with a small amount of aloe vera, such as 1–2 teaspoons, assess your results, and adjust the dose accordingly. Other demulcent herbs are readily available as teas, tablets, and capsules. Supplemental forms, such as slippery elm, licorice, marshmallow, devil's claw, okra, chickweed, comfrey, mullein, plantain, gingko, and corn silk are also available.

Ask Your Doctor

Rule out nutritional deficiencies and anemia. If you have IBD, chronic malabsorption of nutrients—including vitamins D and B12 and folate—is very common, given the nature of the disease and that you may be eating very few foods because you are so uncomfortable. Common nutritional deficiencies in people who have IBD include iron, selenium, vitamins A, B1, B2, B6, C, D, and E, calcium, magnesium, zinc, and folate. Low levels of folate, B12, and B6 can put you at risk for high levels of homocysteine, a major risk factor for deep-vein thrombosis and cardiovascular complications.

CHAPTER 14

Irritable Bowel Syndrome (IBS)

IBS affects nearly 50 million Americans. What is interesting about this syndrome (it's not technically a disease) is that it is defined more by what it is not, rather than what it is. IBS is not an anatomical or structural problem; if you have IBS, everything is just fine with your parts. There is no physical exam, marker on a blood test, or finding on an imaging study that will confirm IBS. In fact, IBS is often diagnosed in the absence of physical and lab findings. IBS is not cancer; it won't cause cancer; and it is not a cause of other gastrointestinal disease.

Motility—the movement of food through your intestines—is the central factor that has gone wrong if you have IBS; it is either too fast or too slow or vacillates between the two. People who have IBS can experience constipation, diarrhea, or a mixture of both that can be cyclical or random. The unpredictability of IBS can also be a source of enormous stress, which can in turn worsen symptoms, creating a feed-forward cycle that is hard to break. Chronic IBS can precipitate other functional gastrointestinal problems such as low digestive capacity and leaky gut.

Gastroenterologists are taught that IBS will be the most common diagnosis they make in their practice, and typically, it has become a self-fulfilling prophecy. Unfortunately, IBS can mimic celiac disease, an even more insidious disease. Savvy doctors will make sure that they rule out this important condition before making a diagnosis of IBS. If you have been diagnosed with IBS but have not been screened for celiac disease, run, do not walk, to your doctor to be tested. Keep in mind that blood tests for celiac disease are not accurate if you have eliminated gluten from your diet. Make sure you have been eating gluten for at least two–three weeks before testing for celiac disease.

This chapter covers a number of other functional issues that are important to rule out if you have been diagnosed with IBS. You owe it to yourself to leave no stone unturned in order to figure out what is really causing your symptoms.

What Does a Diagnosis of IBS Really Tell You?

Not much at all. For one thing, a diagnosis of IBS doesn't tell you where it came from. Some clinicians, however, are eager to hang their hats on stress as the main instigator and don't like to look much farther for any other cause. Many people who suffer from IBS say that when children they were told they had a nervous stomach and still experience anxiety as adults. While chronic stress and anxiety certainly can affect the gastrointestinal tract and speed it up or slow it down, it is only one piece of the puzzle.

When you scratch the surface a little deeper, you'll find that IBS is often a symptom of a dysfunctional gastrointestinal system, rather than something that has sprung up all of a sudden from nowhere.

IBS is multifactorial and unique to the individual, so it is important to become your own detective and assiduously investigate your own body in order find the best approach to control your symptoms or, even better, get at the root of the problem and vanquish it for good.

Food Sensitivities

If you suspect you may have IBS, the first thing to look for is food intolerances and sensitivities. IBS quite often manifests as a result of a long-standing food sensitivity that you were likely not aware of. During the Gut Restoration Program (see page 59), you will be eliminating foods and systematically challenging them, which will give you a very clear idea about which foods work for your body and which cause distress.

Dysbiosis

When your healthy, beneficial bacteria are out of balance with harmful or potentially harmful bacteria, the result is dysbiosis: an imbalance of good guys vs. bad guys. As with inflammatory bowel disease, the links between dysbiosis and IBS are well documented. An enormous population of bacteria live in your large intestine—trillions and trillions of bacterial cells that weigh as much as 4 pounds! These bacteria are so crucial to your well-being that an imbalance can have a body-wide effect.

The beneficial bacteria that live in your gut serve many roles. In particular, they help balance the immune system and regulate peristalsis—the long, slow reflexive wave that our gut uses to get food from our stomach to finally be pooped out. This is quite relevant in the case of IBS.

Your bacteria also protect you from bad, harmful bacteria, and when there's an imbalance, gas, cramping, and bloating—many of the common symptoms of IBS—can result.

Testing for dysbiosis is done with a stool test. Symptoms that you may have dysbiosis include seasonal or recurring diarrhea, frequent or recurring colds, frequent or recurrent kidney, bladder, or vaginal infection, abdominal cramps, and toe or fingernail fungus. Management of dysbiosis typically includes the use of natural antimicrobials, such as garlic, oil of oregano, or berberine, HCl (hydrocholic/stomach acid) and therapeutic doses of probiotics. For the complete protocol, see page 219.

Small Intestine Bacterial Overgrowth (SIBO)

Beneficial bacteria are supposed to be living only in the large intestine. Sometimes, however, even these good guys can end up where they don't belong. If good bacteria creep upstream and set up shop (i.e., fermenting, metabolizing, and doing their bacterial thing) in the small intestine, a disorder called small intestine bacterial overgrowth (SIBO) ensues.

Symptoms that indicate you may have SIBO include

⊚ Excessive gas, bloating, and distension—especially after eating sugar, fiber, and carbohydrates (all of which feed the misplaced bacteria)
⊚ Diarrhea and abdominal pain
⊚ Fibromyalgia syndrome and other complex pain syndromes
  In addition, there is a connection between SIBO and
⊚ Restless legs syndrome (when the legs twitch, move, and burn, especially at night)
⊚ Intolerance to probiotic supplementation
⊚ Low stomach acid and a history of using antacids, proton pump inhibitors, or H2 antagonists

Luckily, SIBO is readily diagnosed with a simple breath test that you can find online or obtain from your doctor. Treatment is actually quite simple and can provide immense relief. Natural antimicrobial substances, such as garlic

compounds or oil of oregano can be used (see page 221 for the complete protocol), but you may opt to take antibiotics concurrently with natural antimicrobial
treatments or follow them with probiotic supplementation. While it may seem
counterintuitive to use an antibiotic in order to fight bacterial overgrowth, it is
much more essential to remove the rogue bacteria—and replenish them in the
right places—than it is to take a rigid stand against antibiotic therapy.

Pathogenic Infection—Candida and Parasites

Infection with a parasite or yeast overgrowth strongly mimics the symptoms of
IBS, and in fact some people who have been diagnosed with IBS have either a
parasite or yeast overgrowth. It is imperative that these infections are ruled out
before making a diagnosis of IBS.

Several years ago, a Candida wave swept the natural and integrative health industry. Every ailment, it seemed, could be pinned to Candida—an overgrowth of yeast.
Everyone was diagnosing Candida, to the extent that it was overdiagnosed. After
a few years of this, the pendulum swung the other way; Candida was dismissed
completely by the medical establishment and doctors who diagnosed patients
with Candida—or even suspected that a patient might have the condition—were
mocked. These days, we understand that while yeast/yeast overgrowth is not present in everyone, it most certainly is in some people, and it is an important condition
to rule out when making a diagnosis of IBS.

Candida, a genus of yeast, is ever present in our world and in our gastrointestinal system. That's right, a small amount of Candida is part of our normal
bacterial flora, but it is kept in check by our good bacteria and a good diet. If it
is allowed to flourish, however, as the result of chronic antibiotic use—or a variety of other factors—that can harm beneficial flora, but not yeast, Candida will
certainly exploit the opportunity to grow. (For more information about Candida,
see page 227.)

As much as you may not like to think about them, parasites are present in the
United States. Parasites are often thought of as little critters that live in faraway,
contaminated lands, but this is not the case. There are several common parasites here in the United States, including *Giardia*, *Blastocystis*, *Cryptosporidium*,
Dientamoeba, *Endolimax*, and *Entamoeba*. These organisms can hang on in your

gastrointestinal system for years and years, making it necessary to develop a keen talent for finding the nearest bathroom, no matter where you happen to be.

There are also worm parasites, which are even less appealing to think about. Hookworms, roundworms, and tapeworms are all found in the United States. Symptoms of worm habitation in your system can include diarrhea, constipation, weight loss, rectal itching, and even blood loss (hookworms feed on blood).

Parasites and Candida overgrowth are readily detected by a comprehensive digestive stool analysis (CDSA). Confirmation with testing rather than self-diagnosis is strongly recommended in order to be precise and targeted with treatment.

Additional Help for IBS

In addition to implementing the Gut Restoration Program (see page 59), there are several additional strategies that you can layer into the program in order to tailor it specifically to your needs.

Dietary Interventions

Emphasize foods that are rich in minerals. This is to help maintain the level of hydration in your cells, which, in turn, helps control how much water you eliminate through your stool. If too much water is eliminated, diarrhea is the result. Your unique sensitivities trump any of our food recommendations (remember, always listen to your body), so with that caveat, try incorporating some of these foods into your diet: leafy greens such as spinach, kale, collards, chard, arugula, and watercress; pumpkin and pumpkin seeds; asparagus; okra; summer squash and zucchini; berries; apples; cherries; coconut; and cocoa (unsweetened and without dairy, of course). Note that cocoa powder could be a problem for some of you. Experiment and assess what works best for you.

Drink up. Water, that is. Adequate water intake—enough to keep your pee a pale, clear yellow—will help alleviate constipation. If you are more prone to diarrhea, hydration is crucial, as you are losing more water than you should be through the stool. If you have chronic diarrhea, or after a bad bout of diarrhea, adding a tiny pinch of salt to a glass of water in the morning will help maintain your electrolyte balance.

Lifestyle Considerations

Do your best to avoid common GI irritants. For anyone who has IBS, caffeine, nicotine, and laxatives (even herbal laxatives) have a negative impact on the motility of the gastrointestinal tract. Although these substances may help with short-term symptom management, they actually exacerbate the underlying motility issue over the long term by creating an overdependence on them, which in turn makes the bowel lazy. If you are using any of these substances, think about using them less often, but go slowly, as quitting cold turkey can have rebound effects, such as even worse constipation.

Chew. Although it seems silly to remind you to chew, wolfing down food while you're standing up introduces a large amount of air into your system that can give you gas pains as it begins to move through your gut. Sit down while you eat and chew your food thoroughly. A trick we like to share with clients is to have them lay their fork down in between bites. This slows down the entire eating process.

Reframing stress. Choosing a positive attitude, showing love, practicing gratitude and appreciation, deep breathing, walking, exercising, and laughing can also begin to calm and soothe the second brain in your gut and lesson IBS symptoms. Biofeedback and other stress-modifying tools can greatly help as well.

Supplements and Herbs

Increase fiber, but remember the golden rule of fiber supplementation. Start low and go slow. In other words, if you are constipated, find a gentle fiber such as acacia or hemp seed and work it slowly into your diet. If you have diarrhea and the mixed type of IBS, acacia and rice bran work well. Start with ½ teaspoon of fiber in 0.24–0.3 liters (8–10 oz.) water for four to five days and make sure you can tolerate that amount. Then, increase to 1 teaspoon of fiber in 0.24–0.3 liters (8–10 oz.) water in the morning and evening. Every five to seven days, increase your fiber by ¼–½ teaspoon per day until you are taking 1 tablespoon of fiber every morning and evening. If you use fiber supplements, it is imperative that you also increase your water intake in order not to become constipated or irritated. Do not add fiber to your diet if you are dehydrated! Stay away from wheat bran and cereals for your fiber sources. Many people who have IBS are also sensitive to wheat, and a recent study indicated that wheat bran made symptoms worse in 55 percent of the participants.

When choosing a probiotic, find one that has *Bifidobacter infantis* strains in it, in addition to *Lactobacillus* and other *Bifidobacter* strains. After you complete the Gut Restoration Program (see page 59), drop your dose down to 20 billion colony-forming units (CFUs).

Consider higher-dose plant enzyme supplementation. During the program, you will be taking plant digestive enzymes with meals. We have had good clinical success with patients who use plant enzymes with their meals and also in between meals, and although we couldn't find studies to back it up, this supplementation works especially well for constipation-type IBS.

Try slippery elm. You can find this herbal remedy in powder, drops, or capsules. We recommend taking several grams daily in divided doses. Slippery elm is a demulcent herb, which means it helps coat, soothe, and lubricate the GI tract. Slippery elm also happens to taste quite delicious.

Peppermint oil. In capsule form, it helps with pain and spasm. A carminative herb, peppermint helps remove gas and reduce cramping, thus greatly reducing gas pains. Take 1–2 capsules on an empty stomach for best results.

Consider ginger. Like peppermint, ginger is great at reducing gas and thus gas pains. You can use fresh or powdered ginger in food, and of course, it is readily available as a tea or crystallized.

Try magnesium glycinate. It works for the constipated type of IBS. Magnesium helps dilate and relax tissues, helping to ease bowel movements. Start with 150–200 milligrams of magnesium glycinate in the form of a capsule or powder before bed, and several days later increase your dose to 300–400 milligrams before bed. If you tolerate that well, take 150 milligrams in the morning and 300–400 milligrams before bed, then work up to 400 milligrams in the morning and before bed. Magnesium is quite safe, but note that if you take too much, it can cause diarrhea.

Vitamin C. Try it for the constipated type of IBS. When taken in high doses, vitamin C is a laxative and stool softener. Everyone has a different level of tolerance for the amount of vitamin C it takes for the laxative effect to kick in. To find your level, start with 500 milligrams twice daily, and double this amount every one to two days. Once you find your vitamin C tolerance level, you may use it on an as-needed basis.

Calcium-magnesium supplement. Try it for diarrhea-dominant IBS. Calcium causes tissue to contract, and you always want to balance this tightening with magnesium, the relaxer. Calcium and magnesium work together to improve the function of the intestines and slow down diarrhea. Find a supplement that has calcium and magnesium in a 2:1 ratio favoring calcium.

Zinc lozenges. These can be used for diarrhea-dominant IBS. You can easily find 5 milligrams zinc lozenges at your local drugstore. You may have 2–3 of these per day, particularly on your bad days.

Carob powder in applesauce. This mixture is an old, natural remedy to slow the bowel, and helps alleviate diarrhea-dominant IBS. Try 1–2 teaspoons of carob powder in 2 tablespoons of applesauce—it really helps.

Serotonin. It is well loved by the enteric nervous system! In fact, there are more serotonin receptors in the gut than there are in the brain, and more of serotonin is produced in the digestive system than anywhere else. The same can be said for many so-called neurotransmitters. Using serotonin-boosting nutrients and amino acids such as 5-HTP, tryptophan, St. John's wort, SAMe, and the like can help soothe and tone an irritated gastrointestinal tract. Next to consider are gamma-aminobutyric acid (GABA)-boosting nutrients and compounds. GABA is the body's major inhibitory/calming/soothing neurotransmitter. It helps everything chill out, including the gut. GABA comes in supplemental form, in blends or alone, typically in capsules. Nutrients and compounds in GABA, such as glycine, L-theanine, and taurine, and herbs such as valerian root, can be taken as an extract or in a capsule. Skullcap and kava kava can also be taken in capsules. There are many herbal and vitamin blends that support neurotransmitter assimilation and receptor sensitivity.

Ask Your Doctor

Dysbiosis, parasites, and Candida infection. These can be ruled out with a comprehensive digestive stool analysis (CDSA). If your doctor will not run this test for you, find one who will! It is that important and could be the key to unlocking your symptoms.

Consider IgG food-allergy testing. A simple blood test can pinpoint food sensitivities. These tests can be ordered by your doctor or through online health companies such as Life Extension.

Parasite Protocol

If you have confirmed parasite infection from a stool test, it's time to send those unwanted passengers packing. Parasites are treated for twelve weeks, in conjunction with the Gut Restoration Program (for the same length of time) to help support the gastrointestinal tract and immune system.

The doses of the therapeutic agents that work against parasites, in the following list, are average recommendations. As always, listen to your body before taking anything. If a dose of any recommended supplement or herb gives you side effects or worsens symptoms, cut the dosage in half or in quarters and go slow. Everyone is different.

It cannot be stressed enough that you must have daily bowel movements before you undertake a parasite protocol. If you have a confirmed parasite and constipation-type IBS, you must get your bowels moving before you initiate this protocol.

The remedies in the following list are best taken on an empty stomach. However, some of them, particularly oil of oregano and garlic, can make you queasy on an empty stomach—definitely not what you want. If they make you feel nauseous, take them with a bit of food.

- *Juglans nigra* (black walnut), *Artemesia absinthium* (wormwood), *Chenopodium ambrosioides* (wormseed) complex: There are many complexes like this available over the counter in capsule or drop form. Take one dose three times daily.
- Berberine: 500 milligrams three times daily, in capsules.
- Oil of oregano: 450 milligrams three times daily.
- Allicin (a powerful compound of garlic): 200 milligrams three times daily.

You may take all four of these remedies at once, or you can start with a couple of them and swap in two of the other antifungals every two to three weeks. This approach may be even more effective than taking all four remedies at once.

CHAPTER 15

Dysbiosis

At its core, dysbiosis is an imbalance between good, beneficial bacteria in your body and potentially harmful, pathogenic organisms. Most of us have a few of these bad guys on board in our digestive tract; but our immune system, the conditions in our gastrointestinal tract, and our microbiota keep them in check.

Antibiotics, acid-blocking drugs, birth control pills, steroids, excessive alcohol consumption, frequent sugar consumption, chronic stress, and the bacterial bad guys themselves can tip the scales to favor the growth of pathogenic organisms, such as harmful bacteria. If you have these bad actors in your system, it does not mean you are going to become violently ill immediately or unable to function, as you would be if you had food poisoning from *Salmonella*. That's because these types of pathogenic organisms are "low virulence." In other words, they don't make you really sick right away. Instead, they create chronic, insidious symptoms that are hard to shake, such as gas, bloating, indigestion, and trouble digesting carbohydrates, fiber, and sugar. Sadly, these symptoms often go unrecognized, undiagnosed, and untreated. This chapter explores the causes of dysbiosis, as well as tests and treatments.

What Is Dysbiosis?

Dysbiosis has been implicated in everything from gas and bloating, diarrhea and constipation, to acne, rashes, headaches, food sensitivities, migraines, stinky breath, indigestion, foul-smelling stool, undigested food in the stool, mucous or blood in the stool, excessive burping, itchiness, urgency to poop, fatigue, and gastritis. It has been linked to celiac disease; interstitial cystitis (IC), in which the lining of the bladder is inflamed and irritated, creating frequent urination, burning with urination, and other symptoms; urinary-tract infection; irritable bowel syndrome (IBS); inflammatory bowel disease (IBD); fibromyalgia and other complex pain syndromes; restless legs syndrome; chronic sinusitis; arthritis; asthma, and auto-immune conditions.

That is quite a list, yet remember that for every human cell, there are ten bacterial cells, which accounts for their ubiquity: dysbiosis can occur in the gastrointestinal tract, but it can also occur in many other places, for example the genitourinary tract (think urinary-tract infections and yeast infections) or in the skin, nails, lungs, sinuses, ears, or eyes, resulting in a range of infections such as athlete's foot and swimmer's ear.

There are a few classes of dysbiosis, and they can overlap. In fact, it is quite common for people to have more than one type of dysbiosis at the same time. The bottom line is dysbiosis is a catchall term for the many ways you can have an imbalance of good and bad bacteria, including

- when you don't have high enough numbers of beneficial bacteria—usually from chronic antibiotic use or from a poor diet that is low in fiber (also known as insufficiency dysbiosis).
- if some of your bacteria move to other parts of the body where they don't belong (i.e., overgrowth dysbiosis). Low stomach-acid production will often cause this, and it is accompanied by gas and bloating. A prime example of this is small intestine bacterial overgrowth (SIBO). (See page 209 for more information about SIBO.) A consequence of this overgrowth is fermentation dysbiosis. Have you ever seen wine being made? Those bubbles are by-products from the bacteria and other organisms in the wine that metabolize and use the sugars and other compounds in the grapes for food. This kind of fermentation is great for folks who enjoy wine, hard cheese, and other fermented foods, but if you have an overgrowth of bacteria in your body you are going to notice a significant increase in gas. It will be worsened by foods that are fermented or high in carbohydrates. Symptoms will improve when you eat foods that are lower in carbohydrates, when you avoid fermented foods, and when you follow the Gut Restoration Program (see page 59) and dysbiosis protocols (see pages 219–221).

Other Types and Causes of Dysbiosis

One of the most common types of dysbiosis is fungal—specifically, Candida infection. Although there are small amounts of Candida present in most of us, it will quickly jump on an opportunity to grow if we give it one. Antibiotics, birth control pills, sugar, and alcohol can offer such chances. Candida is also linked to fermentation dysbiosis and parasitic infection, which is more common in the Western world than we like to think. (See page 210 for more information on parasites.)

◎ By-products of bacteria and yeasts such as Candida can stimulate an inflammatory response from the immune system, which, over time, can lead to leaky gut (see page 26 for more information about leaky gut) and malabsorption of nutrients in the digestive system. In leaky gut, the immune system begins to form antibodies against foods you eat because they are perceived as a threat; and then through a process called molecular mimicry, the immune system may begin making antibodies against your own tissues and spark autoimmune conditions, such as arthritis and multiple sclerosis.

◎ If your body is not producing enough digestive enzymes and acid, and there are insufficient beneficial bacteria, your body's ability to digest protein is impaired. If you can't break down protein, what happens to it? Putrefaction.

◎ Similarly, if you eat a high-protein diet but lack the equipment to break it down, putrefaction dysbiosis will result. This type of dysbiosis can cause vitamin B12 deficiency and has been linked to hormone-related cancers such as prostate, breast, and colon cancer. Luckily, putrefaction dysbiosis can be remediated through the use of supplemental acid, enzymes, and a fiber-rich diet.

Testing for Dysbiosis

◎ **Comprehensive stool analysis.** The best way to see exactly which bacteria have taken up residence in your gut is with a comprehensive digestive stool analysis (CDSA). Various labs offer this kind of test and can give you a broad look at the health and function of your GI tract without being invasive. (See Resources, page 303, for more information about finding a lab near you.) All you have to do is collect a stool sample in the comfort of your own home and send it off to the lab. The lab analyzes the bacteria that live in your gut and identifies any pathogenic bacteria, yeast, or parasite. Your digestive and absorptive functions are measured in terms of pancreatic enzyme output, presence of meat or veggie fibers, and the amount of fats, triglycerides, and cholesterol present in the stool. The lab checks levels of inflammation, along with short-chain fatty-acid production. If you have been dealing with chronic GI issues for a while and have had every other test in the book except this one, it is time to get a comprehensive stool analysis.

◎ **Organic-acid testing.** This test measures compounds in the urine that indicate the presence of pathogenic bacteria or yeast. Organic acids are by-products of metabolism that give us great insight into how effectively the body is working. In addition to giving us a comprehensive view of GI health, organic-acid testing also assesses: vitamin B usage; cellular energy production; neurotransmitter balance and stress; the ability of the body to quench free radicals; and the detoxification capacity of the liver. This test involves collecting a sample of urine at home and then mailing it to a lab for analysis.

◎ **Breath test.** During this test, you drink either a big glass of glucose or lactulose (sugar drinks). Afterward, certain gases in your breath are measured. A rise in hydrogen or methane gas is a good indicator that there is bacterial overgrowth in your small intestine (SIBO). Think of this test as a bacterial Breathalyzer.

◎ **Blood test.** Blood tests can reveal the presence of *H. pylori, Clostridium difficile,* and other opportunistic or potentially harmful bacteria in your body. IgG food-sensitivity tests that show a reaction to brewer's and baker's yeasts should raise suspicions of Candida infection.

Additional Help for Dysbiosis

The variety of natural antimicrobials (agents that stop the growth of micro-organisms, such as bacteria) in the plant world is staggering. These plants, having evolved with us through the millennia, are capable of killing harmful bacteria while sparing the beneficial, friendly bacteria in the GI tract. Natural antimicrobials are very smart hit men and leave little collateral damage. They selectively seek out and kill human pathogens while sparing the bacteria that are beneficial to us.

In stubborn cases of dysbiosis and for anyone who has not been helped by the Gut Restoration Program, pharmaceutical antibiotics could be just the trick.

Remember to double your probiotic intake if you are taking antibiotics, and then take the probiotic for three times the amount of time you were on the antibiotic course. For example, if you have a one-week course of antibiotics, you will take a double dose of probiotics for three weeks. This will help reduce the side effects of antibiotics, i.e., abdominal pain, diarrhea, and C. *difficile* infection, a particularly nasty, and sometimes painful and bloody, type of antibiotic-associated diarrhea. Antibiotics and probiotics don't cancel each other out, and probiotics don't prevent the antibiotic from doing its job.

Dietary Interventions

You can help your body send bad bacteria packing by utilizing a few dietary strategies that decrease favorable conditions for their growth.

Avoid sugar consumption. Remove sugar from your diet until the infection is vanquished. Low glycemic-index fruits such as apples, pears, berries, and cherries are fine, but avoid higher glycemic-index fruits such as grapes, oranges, and tropical fruits such as mango, pineapple, and bananas. Sweets, of course, are off the menu too.

Cook all fibrous food well and start with small amounts. Some types of dysbiosis, such as SIBO, make fiber tough to digest. Listen to your body and don't try to force fiber down. Avoid eating high-fiber vegetables such as raw cabbage, broccoli, and cauliflower (as crudités, for example). Be sure to cook them, along with virtually all other veggies.

Avoid fermented foods. Do not eat these foods for the duration of the Gut Restoration Program as they contain compounds that can enhance the growth of harmful bacteria.

Eat foods that are rich in prebiotics. Prebiotics are fiber compounds that help nourish beneficial bacteria. These include artichoke, asparagus, burdock root, chicory, dandelion, garlic, green tea, raw honey, Jerusalem artichoke (sunchoke), jicama, and onion. These foods should be well cooked, and you should start with small amounts of them.

Here is a good place to remind you that those prebiotic rich foods we've recommended also happen (by the very nature of their carbohydrate profiles) to be rich in FODMAPS (fermentable oligo-di-mono-saccharides and polyols). These types of carbohydrates can cause gas and bloating in some people. So remember to listen to your body.

Herbs and Supplements

The following tried-and-true agents are effective in helping to restore the balance of bacteria in your body:

Allicillin (garlic). Allicillin is an active component of garlic that can kill a wide variety of bacteria, yeast, and parasites. Take 200 milligrams three times daily. Incorporate garlic into your cooking. If you have a difficult time tolerating garlic, listen to your body and use one of the alternatives discussed here.

Oil of oregano. Like garlic, oil of oregano takes action against a variety of pathogens and is highly effective against viruses as well. It is best to find an emulsified oil product that is encapsulated rather than in tablet form. In our experience, encapsulated oil is far more effective. The dose is 200–400 milligrams three times daily.

Grapefruit seed extract (GSE). Highly effective at destroying bacteria, this extract is also powerful against pinworms. The dose is 250 milligrams three times daily.

Probiotics—with a caveat. A high dose of probiotics—upward of 100 billion CFUs—is recommended in the Gut Restoration Program. However, some people may not be able to handle a dose that high. Intolerance to probiotics is a big clue that some type of dysbiosis is present. If this is the case for you, start with a much lower dose, 1–5 billion CFUs, and monitor any symptoms. Each week, try to double your dose, and once again, note any symptoms. If you can't double the dose, that is OK, stay where you are, and try again the next week. As bad bacteria are killed off, you will be able to tolerate higher doses.

CHAPTER 16

Helicobacter pylori and Gastric Ulcer/Gastritis

Helicobacter pylori (*H. pylori*) bacteria are found in the lining of the stomach and affect up to 50 percent of the world's population. Until the discovery of these bacteria in 1982, stress was the main culprit implicated in ulcer formation. The received wisdom at the time was "You'll give yourself an ulcer" if you chain smoke, drink too much coffee, and get stressed out by your job, deadlines, etc. Now, it is known that almost 90 percent of people who have ulcers have an *H. pylori* infection.

H. pylori is a common bacterial infection that can create ulcers and irritation of the stomach and predispose one to certain types of cancers. If you have *H. pylori* and any type of gastrointestinal symptom or disorder, it is important to eradicate this prevalent and pesky invader.

Gastroesophageal reflux disease (GERD), gastritis (inflammation, irritation, or erosion of the stomach lining), and certain stomach cancers can be found with *H. pylori* as well. Infection with *H. pylori* can generate an immune response similar to other types of dysbiosis that ultimately culminates in leaky gut syndrome, a condition in which the lining of the small intestine becomes compromised, leading to abnormal immune signaling, food sensitivity, and malabsorption (the poor absorption of nutrients often due to leaky gut), and a slew of other functional digestive problems. *H. pylori* releases a variety of toxic substances ranging from free radicals, gastrin inhibitors that reduce acid production, various enzymes that break down protective mucous and damage DNA, inflammatory compounds to cytotoxins (toxic compounds that can harm cells) that can kill stomach cells and heat-shock proteins. The result can stimulate a strong immune response, often against the cells of the stomach. In short, *H. pylori* is not a friendly guest.

The Mysteries of *H. pylori*

Since Dr. Barry Marshall stumbled upon *Helicobacter pylori* in the early 1980s, a stampede of researchers has been exploring the ins and outs of this puzzling and seemingly ubiquitous form of bacteria. It has been linked to several diseases, including migraines, psoriasis, rosacea, heart disease, iron-deficiency anemia, vitamin B12–deficiency anemia, interstitial cystitis (IC, a chronic inflammation and irritation of the lining of the bladder leading to bladder pain and urinary frequency), Sjogren's syndrome (an autoimmune condition affecting the glands), Raynaud's phenomenon (a condition in which the microcirculation of the hands and feet causes pain, burning, and discoloration), Parkinson's disease, stomach cancer, colorectal cancer, glaucoma, lichen planus (a condition that forms scabs on skin or in the mouth), and autoimmune thyroid disease.

On the other hand, research suggests that *H. pylori* may offer benefits such as protection against allergies, asthma, eczema, and even inflammatory bowel disease. The hypothesis here is that if you have certain genes, *H. pylori* doesn't affect you as it does others and perhaps even protects you. This begs another question. If so many people have *H. pylori*, why don't all of them have gastrointestinal symptoms? The answer is we just don't know yet. In this way, *H. pylori* is typically treated only if symptoms are present, such as an ulcer, gastritis, unremitting iron-deficiency anemia, stomach cancer, or suspicious-looking lesions in the stomach.

Conventional Treatment of *H. pylori*

Triple or quadruple antibiotic therapy is the conventional treatment of *H. pylori*. Triple therapy requires that you take two antibiotics plus a proton pump inhibitor for two weeks. Quadruple therapy calls for bismuth subsalicylate, another medicinal compound that targets *H. pylori* in addition to triple therapy. Side effects of these treatments are common and include diarrhea and stomach pain, headache, dark stools, and sensitivity to alcohol and sunlight. Relapse rates range from 10 to 20 percent.

There are additional problems with triple and quadruple therapy, not the least of which is that *H. pylori* easily becomes resistant to antibiotics, and consequently, they can only be used once. Another problem with these therapies is that proton inhibitors suppress acid production. Research has suggested that acid blockers can aid in the healing of ulcers, but on the flip side, they increase rates of antibiotic resistance and may worsen gastritis! Ultimately, it is up to you and your doctor to determine if triple or quadruple therapy is right for your situation. These therapies certainly should be considered if natural remedies have not been effective for you. Just remember to double the dose of probiotics you're taking throughout your antibiotic course, and then continue to take a double dose of probiotics for three times as long as the antibiotic course (for example, one week of antibiotics equals three weeks of doubled-up probiotics). Double dosing probiotics will help prevent and offset any side effects from the antibiotics.

Additional Help for *H. pylori*

These interventions can be done in conjunction with pharmaceutical therapy. Each one of them is useful and not contraindicated with conventional antibiotic treatment.

Dietary Interventions

These simple dietary interventions will actually help the lining of your stomach heal faster!

Cabbage. Find ways to work cabbage—cooked cabbage, raw cabbage, cabbage juice, sauerkraut, etc.—into your life. It wants to be there to help you fight *H. pylori*. In fact, there is a long history of using cabbage to treat ulcers and stomach complaints, the significant benefits of which have been borne out in current research. Aim for 1–2 cups daily.

Brussels Sprouts and Other Cruciferous Vegetables. Brussels sprouts and broccoli and their sprouts, kale, cauliflower, and bok choi are rich in the sulfur-containing amino acid methionine (cabbage is also in this family). This amino acid is very effective in the fight against *H. pylori* and promotes tissue healing. Incorporate several one-cup servings weekly. If you have difficulty digesting these foods, cook them well and start with small amounts.

Onions. Rich in the bioflavonoid quercetin, onions help quash free radicals and reduce inflammation, and when they are cooked, onions have a slippery quality that soothes irritated tissue. Have several servings of cooked onions weekly.

Cinnamon. Sprinkle this slippery, demulcent herb on fruit and find other ways to incorporate it into your diet and hot drinks.

Garlic. A powerful antimicrobial that works against many strains of bacteria, parasites, and yeast, garlic is an ingredient that should be incorporated into your diet every day. If you can tolerate it, chew some raw garlic cloves when you have meals. The raw stuff is definitely not for everyone—especially if you're going out on a first date—so you can use 200 milligrams of Allicillin, twice a day, instead.

Green tea. Humble green tea has been shown to slow the growth of *H. pylori*. We recommend that you drink green tea as often as you like, if you tolerate it well. It is delicious warm or iced.

Supplements and Herbs

Many of these herbs and supplements have been used successfully for centuries. Now their benefits have been borne out in current scientific literature.

Mastic. A resin from a tree native to Greece, mastic has a long historic of use in stomach disorders and stomach pain. The dose is 500 milligrams twice daily, with or without food.

Deglycyrrhizinated licorice (DGL). A soothing and calming herb, licorice helps relieve ulcers by coating irritated tissues, thus protecting them from stomach acid. Try 750 milligrams of DGL twice daily, taken after meals.

Zinc carnosine. This supplement helps to regenerate the lining of the stomach and small intestine, while protecting the lining of the stomach from ulceration and the irritating effects of stomach acid. Zinc carnosine is a major player in the Gut Restoration Program (see page 59). If you have an ulcer, the dosage for zinc carnosine should be increased to 150 milligrams twice daily.

Methylsulfonylmethane (MSM). A compound derivative of the sulfur-containing amino acid methionine, MSM is found in high amounts in cabbage and other vegetables in the cabbage family. Raw cabbage, particularly raw cabbage juice, has been studied extensively in the eradication of *H. pylori* and the cure for ulcers. If you don't feel like drinking a quart of raw cabbage juice every day, MSM is for you. Take 100–200 milligrams twice a day.

Vitamin C. High vitamin C intake has been shown to help reduce the risk of infection with *H. pylori*, eradicate infection, and heal tissue. Vitamin C is also one of the building blocks of collagen and, thus, can help rebuild our soft tissues—including that of the digestive tract. The dose is 500 milligrams twice daily.

Vitamin E. Like vitamin C, vitamin E been shown to protect against *H. pylori* infection. Research suggests that supplementation with mixed tocopherols (vitamin E) aids in destroying *H. pylori*. Infection with *H. pylori* generates free radicals, and vitamin E, as an antioxidant, is one of our best defenses. Take 400 IU mixed tocopherols daily.

Aloe. There are two ways to take aloe as a supplement to fight *H. pylori*—as a juice or as a powder that has been dehydrated at low temperature to maintain the active compounds found in the juice. Take 500 milligrams of aloe two to three times daily, after meals. If you plan to take the juice, take an ounce after meals. Like the sap squeezed from an aloe leaf, the juice is soothing and calming to irritated tissues and can help reduce pain.

Grapefruit seed extract (GSE). Take 10 drops of this liquid concentrate, a natural compound derived from the seed and pulp of grapefruit, three times daily. GSE has strong antimicrobial action. A few years ago, researchers found that many commercial brands were adulterated with synthetic antimicrobials, including benzethonium chloride (which has not been approved for use in the United States as a food additive). Make sure that the product you buy, from a reputable source, has been vetted for purity.

CHAPTER 17

Candida

Candida overgrowth is a special form of dysbiosis. Since *Candida albicans* (meaning "white," the color of this yeast) belongs in the yeast family, it is referred to as a yeast infection.

Candida is ubiquitous. Most of us have some Candida on our skin or inside of us. In small amounts, Candida is harmless and can actually assist our beneficial gut flora—the same friendly bacteria that, along with the immune system, keep Candida populations small and in check. When that balance is lost and Candida is able to overgrow and take over, it can wreak havoc on the whole body.

An Opportunistic Critter

The gastrointestinal and genitourinary tracts are like huge parking lots. All of the parking spaces should be filled with good guys—beneficial bacteria. If for some reason your beneficial bacteria population dips or is compromised, spaces are left for Candida to move in and multiply. Because it is opportunistic by nature, Candida will not miss a chance to exploit a weakness whenever it can.

Antibiotic use, overconsumption of alcohol and sugar, chronic stress, steroid use, and birth control pills can be harmful to beneficial bacteria, decreasing their population and creating a chance for Candida to take hold and multiply quickly.

Good bacteria also use estrogen and progesterone as one of their sources of food and, as women enter the week before menses, they can be prone to yeast and bladder infections. As hormone levels decline during the week before bleeding (indeed, it is these declining levels that trigger bleeding) the good bacterial population dips, and Candida multiplies to fill in the empty spaces. This is why many women report yeast or bladder infections before menses. If this sounds like you, you will find that the Gut Restoration Program (see page 59) will help you significantly, because it makes your beneficial bacterial populations more robust and creates unfavorable conditions for Candida to thrive.

The Great Pretender

When there is Candida overgrowth in the GI tract, it can spell trouble for the whole body. As a natural by-product of its metabolism, Candida produces compounds that are inherently harmful to our bodies—similar compounds are found in nail polish remover!

Symptoms of Candida overgrowth mimic many other conditions and symptoms, which is why it is important to confirm or deny the presence of overgrowth with testing (for example, a comprehensive digestive stool analysis, organic-acid test, or blood test). In fact, up to one-fifth of people diagnosed with Irritable Bowel Syndrome (IBS) actually have Candida overgrowth, and when treated, IBS disappears. For this reason, Candida has been referred to as the great pretender.

Symptoms of Candida overgrowth include gas and bloating; belly pain; intestinal pain; constipation; diarrhea; exhaustion; muscle aches; foggy thinking; anxiety and depression; sensitivity to smells, sounds, and light; insomnia; tinnitus; allergies; blood-sugar issues; toenail infection/athlete's foot; bladder infection; vaginal infection; itchiness; food intolerance, etc. Symptoms tend to be worse on muggy and wet days or in places where there is mold.

A major consequence of Candida overgrowth is the production of compounds that damage the lining of the small intestine and whip the immune system into a dysfunctional inflammatory state. Leaky gut develops in this perfect storm of inflammation, which leads to the release of even more inflammatory compounds (by the immune system) and an ever-expanding list of food sensitivities, as the immune system begins to make antibodies against everything you eat.

Additional Help for Candida

There are several medications and natural substances that help kill Candida, but herbs and other compounds will not work unless your diet is calibrated to support healing. For some, the diet plan from the Gut Restoration Program (see page 59) will be enough to help greatly. Others may have to further reduce the number of carbohydrates and sugars in their diet. It is important to experiment to find what works best with you. Start with the diet recommendations on page 229 first. Try it for two weeks, and if your symptoms don't improve, you may want to consider restricting carbohydrates even more.

When it comes to herbal anti-Candida agents, it is best to start at a low dose and slowly increase the dosage in order to reduce the symptoms of Candida as it dies off. Here's why: As Candida die, they release proteins and various endotoxins that can make you feel tired and headachy and actually worsen symptoms.

Dietary Interventions

The key to treating Candida overgrowth is to starve them of their most beloved food: sugar. There are a variety of Candida diets out there, and they all emphasize low-carbohydrate intake. Vegetables, proteins, and healthy fats should be the base of the diet. Sugars, all grains, caffeine, and most fruits should be eliminated for the course of treatment. These two diets are recommended:

www.thecandidadiet.com

www.gapsdiet.com

Coconut oil and other coconut products. Coconut has powerful anti-Candida properties and adds fuel to your GI system, helping to speed healing. Plus, coconut tastes delicious! You can use coconut oil in smoothies or to sauté veggies, and you can also rub it into your skin (it's a great moisturizer).

Water. Adequate water intake cannot be overstated while you are on a Candida elimination protocol. Aim for at least 3 liters (5 pints) of clean, filtered water daily. Caffeine-containing products do not count toward this amount.

Lifestyle Interventions

A few simple steps—such as improving your diet, getting more sleep, and reducing stress—can go a long way toward eradicating Candida. In addition to those important lifestyle changes, try some of these to help put the kibosh on the growth of Candida:

Dry brushing. This is beneficial for reducing symptoms of Candida overgrowth and to keep you feeling great during the course of the Gut Restoration Program (see page 59). Every day, before you shower, brush your entire body with a dry loofah or soft-bristled body brush. Use short, firm strokes until your skin is lightly flushed—there's no need to scrape or use a lot of pressure. Always remember to brush toward your heart, starting from your fingertips, and then moving on to your torso and legs, beginning with your toes.

Infrared sauna therapy. The sauna also eases any die-off symptoms of Candida. Start with just a few minutes of sitting in the sauna to make sure you can tolerate it, and then slowly increase the time, up to 20 minutes. Because the sauna helps eliminate waste products through the skin (a major organ of detoxification), always shower afterward so that they are not reabsorbed.

Sleep. Adequate sleep—7 hours at a bare minimum—is crucial for the restoration of gut health and to aid your immune system in fighting off a Candida infection. Make sure that your bedroom is dark and cool for optimal sleep. Electronics—particularly your television, laptop, tablet, and cell phone—stacks of bills, and work-related paperwork, should not be in your sleeping space. Sleep should be as high a priority for you as excellent nutrition and drinking plenty of water.

Supplements and Herbs

There are a wide variety of natural antifungal agents that work to knock back yeast infections. Try some of these:

Allicillin (garlic). Garlic is an antimicrobial that inhibits the growth of many different strains of bacteria, from parasites to Candida and pathogenic bacteria. Start with 200 milligrams once daily for one week, then increase the dose to 200 milligrams twice daily and monitor symptoms. If you tolerate this well, take up to 200 milligrams three times daily.

Oil of oregano. Try taking 450 milligrams once daily for one week, then increase the dose to 450 milligrams twice daily and monitor symptoms. If you are feeling good and symptoms are not being exacerbated, increase the dose once again to 450 milligrams three times daily. If at any time you begin to feel bad—headache, body ache, fatigue, etc.—drop down to a lower dose. (Remember that these are symptoms of yeast die-off—the very thing you want to accomplish, but as you start to kill the yeast, their bodies release toxins that can be harmful and make you feel bad temporarily.)

Saccharomyces boulardii. *Sacchromyces boulardii* is a type of yeast. You might be thinking, "Why on Earth would you use yeast to kill yeast?" Though it is true that both *Saccharomyces* and *Candida* are yeasts, each is a unique species with different actions, preferences, and food sources. Similarly, though cats and mice are both mammals, cats hunt and kill mice, nevertheless. Consider *S. boulardii* to be the cat of the yeast world, and *Candida* the mouse. Take 5 billion organisms of *S. boulardii* (if that is how the product is designated) or 250 milligrams, twice daily.

Ask Your Doctor

Sometimes, natural antifungals may not be enough to eradicate Candida infection. If this is the case, your doctor can prescribe a course of a drug called nystatin, a pharmaceutical antifungal that is great at destroying yeast infections of the gut. Because it is not usually absorbed into the general circulation of the body, it is typically well tolerated by most people.

CHAPTER 18

Asthma

According to the Centers for Disease Control and Prevention (CDC), asthma is on the rise in a big way. Newly reported cases of asthma increased by more than 4 million between 2001 and 2009. Currently, almost 19 million adults in the United States—one in twelve—have asthma, while one in ten children—a total of 7.1 million kids—struggle with this disease. The largest rate of increase in the last decade has been in African American and inner-city children. When you tally the cost of drugs, hospital visits, and missed work, we spend a whopping $60 billion per year on asthma. It's enough to take your breath away. With a price tag this high, it is almost intuitive that, if there are things in our environment and diet that we can control to help us reduce the frequency and severity of attacks, we should jump on the opportunity.

If you're wondering what a chapter on asthma is doing in a book about digestion, the answer is quite simple. Asthma, at its core, is driven by changes in the immune system that create inflammation in the airways, thus making them more clogged and more difficult for air to flow through. Because the seat of the immune system is the gut—where more than two-thirds of the immune system resides—an intuitive step to take is optimizing gut health and immune function through the Gut Restoration Program (see page 59).

What Is Asthma and Where Does It Come From?

Asthma is a condition of the airways that creates wheezing, shortness of breath, and difficulty breathing that ranges from mild to life threatening. Asthma can be triggered by exercise, pollutants in the environment, stress, or nothing at all. The high—and increasing—rate of asthma in the United States has led researchers and epidemiologists to look for answers and novel approaches for treatment. The development of asthma has many factors including repeated environmental exposure to triggers such as allergens, pollutants, foods, microbes, and even stress.

Several studies have linked food to asthma and indicate that inner-city children who don't have access to omega-3-rich foods are at an increased risk for asthma.

Studies have also shown the correlation between the presence of IgG antibodies in the body and asthma. A diet high in allergenic foods such as bread, sugar, grain, dairy products, fake fats, soy, etc., increases the production of IgG antibodies. Over time, this accelerated production will set the stage for chronic disease, including asthma. The exact mechanisms have not been fully teased out, but proof that low-allergen diets help mitigate symptoms of asthma is piling up.

Additional Help for Asthma

There are several steps you can take to help soothe the symptoms of asthma through nutrition, as well as targeted supplementation and some changes you can make around the house.

Dietary Interventions

A few key concepts have come out of recent research into the connection between nutrition and asthma. The bottom line? The food you eat—and don't eat—can greatly impact the way you breathe.

Increase vegetable intake. This is especially important for children (and their rapidly developing immune systems). Veggies are packed with airway-soothing compounds and free-radical-fighting antioxidants. If you feel daunted by the task of keeping fresh produce in the fridge, buy frozen veggies (they're just as good as the fresh stuff).

Consider long-term avoidance of allergenic foods. Gluten, dairy, and soy are highly stimulating to the immune system in a potentially dysfunctional way because they generate antibody production that can drive asthma. Low-allergen diets help reduce the intensity and number of asthma attacks.

Consider long-term avoidance of foods that increase mucous production. The main foods that crank up your mucous factory are wheat, milk, orange juice, and sugar. This may seem like a random list, but these foods have risen to the top of the mucous-producing pile. No more cereal with orange juice for breakfast if you want to breathe better.

Lifestyle Interventions

You have little control over the environment outside of your home, but you do have control over the environment inside it. These strategies are all aimed at cleaning up your environment and will greatly improve the air quality of your home by removing factors that can overstimulate the immune system and worsen asthma symptoms.

Invest in a high-quality air filter. Reducing exposure to all irritants and allergens is a cornerstone strategy to decreasing asthma symptoms. Indoor air quality is notoriously poor. If you don't ventilate your house (incredibly, many allergists and immunologists actually suggest that you don't!) the air becomes more concentrated with dust, dirt, mites, dander, and whatever you track in with your shoes. An air filter can help remove these. Check out www.IQair.com for information on top-notch filters. We recommend ventilating your house for 10 minutes every day and using an air filter, at least in your bedroom.

Vacuum and dust regularly. Removing allergens from your environment gives your immune system less stuff to react to. Let's face it, these chores can be a total bore, but by completing them at least once a week (or paying someone to do it for you!), you can keep your immune system calm and reduce asthma symptoms.

Wash bedding in hot water once a week. Routine washing of bedclothes cuts down your exposure to dust mites and their excrement, a major irritant. Have you ever seen one of those close-up pictures of dust mites? Once you get a good look, you will happily throw your sheets into the wash. For an added bonus, use non-chlorine bleach. Bleach is a major airway irritant, so it is important to seek out the versions that don't include chlorine.

Consider instituting a "no shoes in the house" rule. Remembering to take your shoes off, especially if you and your family are used to wearing shoes in the house, can take some doing, but if you live in an urban environment, consider what you are tracking into your home. For one thing, car exhaust settles onto roads and sidewalks, which you then track into your house on your shoes. Other offenders, conventional fertilizers used in landscaping, are heavily contaminated with lead, and of course, the stuff falls off your shoes when you walk into the house. These irritants get stirred into the air you breathe and subsequently stimulate your immune system if your house is unventilated and you don't use an air purifier.

Get rid of carpeting ASAP. Even a carpet that is vacuumed and cleaned regularly still harbors dozens of pounds of dust, dust mites, dander, skin flakes, particulates, and other stuff floating around your house. One of the best investments you can make for your long-term health is getting rid of carpeting and installing hardwood, laminate, or tile flooring, and using throw rugs that you can wash.

Supplements and Herbs

As you clean up your home and external environment, you can also begin to work on your insides with targeted supplementation that reduces inflammation, soothes the immune system, and relaxes the airways.

Fish oil. Consider long-term supplementation with fish oil, which helps the body decrease the creation of inflammatory compounds called leukotrienes that can trigger and exacerbate asthma symptoms. Adults can take 2–4 grams of fish oil combined EPA and DHA. Kids should take 400–500 milligrams combined EPA and DHA.

Bromelain. Bromelain is an enzyme taken from the stem of pineapple. It is a powerful antioxidant and helps dissolve mucous. The dose is 500 milligrams three times daily, preferably between meals, on an empty stomach.

Probiotics. Probiotics are a major component of the Gut Restoration Program (see page 59), and people with asthma should stay on them indefinitely. You can reduce your dose after the program to between 5–20 billion CFUs per day.

Antioxidant supplements. Free-radical damage is a big-time consequence of asthma, which increases inflammation in the body even further. To quench inflammation and free-radical damage and calm it down, look for a product that has a wide variety of antioxidants, including fat-soluble vitamins A and E, vitamin C, bioflavanoids, selenium, and zinc.

Magnesium glycinate. Magnesium is the quintessential relaxer. It helps open up airways and loosen muscles. If you have asthma, take 150 milligrams of magnesium glycinate 20 minutes before exercising. This will help decrease the reactivity of your airways when you exercise, helping it to not tighten up and lowering mucous production. You can also take 150–400 milligrams before bed. Note that if you use too much magnesium too quickly, it can have a laxative effect, so build slowly.

N-acetyl cysteine (NAC). This nutritional supplement acts like nature's Mucinex. It helps thin mucous, making it less likely to block your airways. It also is one of the building blocks to glutathione, one of the most powerful antioxidants made by the body. NAC helps quell inflammation, and as a side benefit, it is fabulous for the liver and helps offset the negative effects of injectable dyes used in contrast (CT/CAT) scans. Take 200 milligrams 1–3 times daily.

Ask Your Doctor

Everyone with asthma should have an IgG food-allergy test to rule out food sensitivities. Remember, IgG sensitivities are responsible for chronic symptoms and are different from IgE allergies, which create immediate, sometimes life-threatening reactions. It is important to note that many people with asthma also have IgE allergies, for which they may have received allergy shots. People with asthma are more prone to allergies, which it is why they should also explore for IgG-type sensitivity.

CHAPTER 19

Arthritis

Arthritis is a broad term for inflamed and achy joints. The most common forms of arthritis are osteoarthritis (OA) and rheumatoid arthritis (RA), although there are many other types of arthritis and conditions that are associated with arthritis (any suggestions for treatment and symptom management in this chapter apply to those as well). This chapter explores the ins and outs—the symptoms and causes as well as potential means of relief—of joint pain.

Osteoarthritis (OA)

Osteoarthritis is usually attributed to the aging and overuse of joints, but it would be a huge oversight to conclude that diet and lifestyle have no influence on this common musculoskeletal affliction. Many savvy practitioners contend that nutritional insufficiencies, chronic inflammation, and a sedentary lifestyle worsen OA. Others have linked OA to food sensitivities. This is why it is necessary to discover which foods your body is uniquely sensitive to, and which ones spark flare-ups. The elimination and challenge portion of the Gut Restoration Program (see page 59) will help you identify exactly which foods, if any, make your joints feel worse.

Non-steroidal anti-inflammatory drugs (NSAIDs) are the primary drug of choice for the management of osteoarthritis. They help reduce pain, of course, but they come with a price. NSAIDs compromise the lining of the GI tract, making it susceptible to ulcers, gastritis, and leaky gut—all well-known side effects of chronic NSAID use. In addition, the body's ability to repair soft tissue is impaired by chronic use of these drugs—an irony because OA is, in part, characterized by degraded soft tissue.

Rheumatoid Arthritis (RA)

Rheumatoid arthritis is an autoimmune condition in which the immune system destroys the synovial fluid in joints—your elbow or knee, for example—and leaves red, swollen, painful joints in its wake. RA lends itself well to the Gut Restoration Program (see page 59) because it may uncover a long-standing case of leaky gut and immune dysfunction that needs to be addressed. As an auto-immune disease, the root of RA is a dysfunctional immune response to the body's own tissue, which can stem from and worsen from issues in the digestive tract related to leaky gut. In leaky gut, the lining of the small intestine becomes compromised. That lining is the interface between the immune system and the food we eat. When that integrity is breached, the immune system can actually make antibodies against those foods! If this goes on long enough, the immune system can "make the leap" and begin making antibodies against its own tissue in a process known as molecular mimicry.

Treatment for RA includes NSAIDs and a cocktail of other drugs such as steroids, immunosuppressive drugs, TNF-alpha inhibitors, and disease-modifying antirheumatic drugs—all of which come with serious side effects. Steroids in particular are difficult on the gut, and using them over the long term can contribute to leaky gut. As a consequence, the immune system steps up production of inflammatory molecules and antibodies, resulting in an escalating cascade of inflammation and an ever-worsening dysfunctional immune response.

Additional Help for Arthritis

Movement is not just necessary to everyday activities and work, it is a joyous expression of life; and when that movement is curtailed by joint pain, it is no fun at all! The following strategies are designed to help you move with greater ease and help reduce other symptoms of joint pain.

Dietary Interventions

The following symptom treatments suggested can be done in conjunction with pharmaceutical management of OA and RA. The goals are to reduce pain and inflammation and support soft tissue repair.

Carefully reintroduce "sensitive" foods. During the Gut Restoration Program (see page 59), you will eliminate certain foods for a time and then reintroduce them one by one—and several days apart—into your diet. Giving yourself a break between eating particular foods you might be sensitive to lets you fully assess their impact on your health and pinpoint the ones that trigger symptoms. In all types of arthritis, there is a strong connection between pain and stiffness and food sensitivity. So, pay attention to foods that may be hurting you.

Increase fish consumption. Fish is a great source of protein, which the body uses to build and repair soft tissue in your joints. Cold-water fish such as salmon, halibut, mackerel, tuna, and sardines are rich in anti-inflammatory omega-3 fatty acids.

Consider long-term elimination of nightshades. Nightshades are relevant to arthritis in two major ways. The first is that nightshades contain compounds that can exacerbate leaky gut, a major concern for people with RA and other autoimmune conditions. The second consideration is that about 15 percent of all people with arthritis are quite sensitive to nightshades, and nightshade elimination greatly improves symptoms. For people with OA, we recommend watching the reintroduction of nightshades to see how they make you feel. If you have RA, we recommend permanent elimination of the nightshade family (tomatoes, white potatoes, eggplant, bell pepper, chili pepper).

Incorporate anti-inflammatory herbs. Ginger, *Boswellia*, devil's claw, and garlic are available as whole ingredients—in the case of ginger and garlic—as well as supplements in a variety of forms and can easily be used in cooking and teas.

Lifestyle Interventions

The goal of these suggestions is to get you moving more—and moving more freely.

Move. Movement is life. Incorporate walks, stretching, and strength training into your everyday life. If you haven't been exercising, start really slowly. A ten-minute walk once or twice a week is better than zero walks per week. Exercise does not have to be all or nothing, but it is crucial for joint mobility. Walking and strength training release anti-inflammatory and antiaging compounds, helping you to feel better. They also help balance the "fight or flight" and "rest and digest" branches of the nervous system. Movement is an underutilized medicine and is completely free of charge. Although people with painful joints may be reluctant to walk, the movement itself can actually help them feel better through the release of anti-inflammatory compounds.

Try topical capsicum cream. This cream is made from cayenne pepper. It is great for temporary relief and is widely available over the counter. Research has shown that capsicum cream is so effective it helps up to 50 percent of people who suffer from arthritis. It is a great go-to remedy to get you through bad days. Heads up: it may sting a bit when first applied. It is, after all, cayenne pepper.

Supplements and Herbs

Many, many supplements and herbs help reduce swelling, pain, and inflammation and help repair damaged joints and tissues. These are some of the superstars:

Curcumin. Curcumin is one of the most powerful natural NSAIDs available. It blocks every inflammatory molecule found in the body and has applications not just for pain reduction but also for brain health, cancer prevention and treatment, chronic illness, and inflammatory bowel conditions, to name just a few. In other words, it is simply a blockbuster, and luckily, it can be found just about everywhere. You will be hearing a lot about curcumin in the years to come. We strongly recommend that you find a curcumin product that is bound to a phosopholipid to improve absorption into the bloodstream and bioavailability. Meriva and BCM-95 preparations are bound to phosphatidylcholine and can be sourced through your health-care provider or online. Take 2 grams twice daily.

Bromelain. Bromelain is an enzyme derived from the stems of pineapple. Don't use bromelain if you have sensitivity to pineapple. Bromelain can be very effective for arthritic pain, but the trick is to take it on an empty stomach at a fairly high dose. We recommend 1.5 grams two to three times daily, in between meals. Bromelain helps reduce inflammation by slowing down the production of pro-inflammatory molecules. Bromelain also helps thin the blood and improve immune function. If you take it with food, it acts as a digestive aid.

Fish oil. Fish oil contains anti-inflammatory compounds that reduce pain and swelling and confer mobility to the joints. Aim for 2–4 grams of combined EPA and DHA—the main constituents of fish oil. For quality reasons, it is important that amounts of these constituents are listed on the label so you know how much you are getting. Run the other way from a product that says only "fish oil: 2 grams per serving." If you get the "fish burps," you may want to get a better-quality supplement or try putting your capsules in the freezer and taking them before bed. (Freezing reduces rancidity, making it a lot easier to take these fishy supplements, and prolongs freshness.) For over-the-counter brands, Nordic Naturals and Carlson's are excellent quality.

Vitamin C. Vitamin C wears a lot of hats when it comes to arthritis support. It helps your body make collagen and boosts soft tissue production. It is a famous anti-inflammatory compound and free-radical quencher, helping to clear excessive inflammation in the body. It helps balance immune response, making the immune system less reactive and helping to protect against bacteria and yeasts that may exacerbate pain and inflammation. Start with 500 milligrams twice daily.

Glucosamine sulfate. Glucosamine sulfate can help build and replenish cartilage and reduce pain. It needs to be taken for at least six weeks to assess efficacy. The dose is 1,500 milligrams three times daily.

Chondroitin. Chondroitin, like glucosamine sulfate, helps to rebuild and repair soft tissue and increase mobility. Give it at least twelve weeks of consistent supplementation to see how it affects the way you feel. Dose is 200–400 milligrams twice daily. Often chondroitin and glucosamine sulfate are found together in products.

MSM. MSM is a sulfur-rich compound with anti-inflammatory and antioxidant properties. It donates sulfur compounds to the body for collagen production and acts against parasites, asthma, and allergies. MSM is best absorbed when taken with vitamin C. Take 1 gram with your vitamin C twice daily.

Multivitamin/multi-mineral complex. Building healthy bone and soft tissue is no small feat, and your body could use all the support it can get. Unfortunately, the mineral content of the soil in which we grow our food is diminishing with every generation, much to the detriment of the nutrient content of the foods we eat. Luckily for us—and especially for those who have arthritis—multivitamins and minerals help fill dietary gaps with dozens of the nutrients required for optimal production of bone and soft tissues.

B complex with folate. Folate is readily available to the body, in contrast to folic acid, which the body has to convert into "active folate." Some people lack the ability to turn folic acid into folate in a genetic abnormality called the MTHFR gene mutation (see page 46). People with this mutation are susceptible to depression, thyroid issues, high homocysteine (a condition that can increase cardiovascular risk), and various kinds of anemia (i.e., pernicious anemia and vitamin B anemia), as well as arthritis.

Ask Your Doctor

If you have arthritis, particularly RA, you may want to have your IgG food sensitivities checked, in case you are eating a food that is overstimulating your immune system. Finding out which foods you are sensitive to, beyond those that are eliminated during the Gut Restoration Program (see page 59), can further help healing.

Ask your health-care provider to check for the MTHFR gene mutation. People with this mutation cannot convert folic acid into active folate, putting them at risk for a variety of health conditions, including arthritis. If you have arthritis and the gene mutation, taking folate will be a major component of your treatment.

CHAPTER 20

Metabolic Damage/ Weight Loss Resistance

You may be wondering what gastrointestinal health has to do with weight loss resistance. As it turns out, the two have quite a lot to do with one another because your digestive system communicates and interacts with every other body system every day. As such, it has a major impact on what your hormonal system is doing, which in turn has a huge effect on whether you are getting fatter or leaner. When the wrong types of habits are cultivated for too long, changes in the nervous, digestive, and hormonal systems that favor weight gain can kick in, making it difficult to lose weight. If you have been struggling to lose weight to no avail, the key just may be in your gut.

Your Nervous System: Stressing vs. Chilling

Your nervous system is divided into two main branches. The sympathetic, or "fight or flight," branch is responsible for releasing stress hormones that get your body ready to head for the hills when you are in danger or have to fight for your life. These days, we don't have to face dangerous, fanged predators lying in wait for us in the grass. Instead, a long list of other stressors put us in fight or flight mode before we even catch a glimpse of a tiger, real or imaginary. Do any of these scenarios sound familiar? Getting stressed while you're stuck in traffic; suffering from a lack of sleep; fighting with family (or anyone else); and bottling up the anger and frustration you feel about your boss, job, or perhaps your marriage; etc. Chronic calorie deprivation, yo-yo dieting, and excessive cardiovascular exercise (such as jogging) may not be immediately recognizable as stressors, but they too hold huge sway over the sympathetic nervous system.

The parasympathetic nervous branch, on the other hand, is known as the "rest and digest" arm of the nervous system. It helps you relax, chill out, and feel mellow. It keeps your road rage in check and helps you hold your tongue when you want to snap at someone. It ensures proper digestive function and helps the brain orchestrate hormonal balance. Without good parasympathetic nervous-system function, you can be more prone to tummy aches, acid reflux, indigestion, diarrhea, and other digestive disturbances. Over time, digestion can become impaired, resulting in malabsorption of nutrients, excessive inflammation in the digestive tract, and even leaky gut.

The Downside of Chronic Dieting and Overexercising

The sympathetic and parasympathetic branches of the nervous system are always in relative balance, like a seesaw. But . . . guess what? If you are chronically on a low-calorie diet and exercise to excess, doing so will begin to tip the seesaw toward the sympathetic nervous system. When you allow this imbalance to persist for months and years, you are paving the way to sympathetic dominance—as if you have an elephant sitting on one end of your nervous system and a Chihuahua on the other. By this time, you will have noticed that what used to work before isn't working now, and you are not losing any weight. In fact, you may even be gaining some weight, in spite of your efforts. On top of all that, you are probably noticing that you are

- feeling tired and sluggish
- not thinking clearly
- more sensitive to light
- losing some hair, and your skin may not look as good as it used to
- taking longer to recover from injuries and workouts
- catching colds more frequently
- experiencing a low libido
- experiencing GI symptoms that you never had before—bloating, burping, and burning
- experiencing premenstrual symptoms that you have not had previously
- no longer menstruating

Metabolic Dominoes

To describe the phenomenon of cascading symptoms that result when the sympathetic and parasympathetic branches of the nervous system are out of whack, Dr. Jade Teta coined the term *metabolic dominoes*. Here's how they affect each other:

- Chronic stress from overdieting and too much cardio create sympathetic dominance in the nervous system, which irritates the brain, the way a fly does when it keeps buzzing in your ear. In the short term, this level of stress is manageable, but over time, it creates an environment in which the brain becomes so irritated that it floods the thyroid, adrenal, and reproductive organs with signals that they should start increasing activity. Hormones released from the brain that control the thyroid, adrenal, and reproductive organs increase—at least in the short term—and adrenaline, a major stress hormone, increases. The body is able to compensate for elevation of stress and increased hormone production for a while, but then the receptors for these stress hormones become "down regulated" (i.e., cells "pull in" the receptors that "hear" the message, and our physiology struggles to hear their message). This activity is like whipping a tired horse. The brain, adrenal, thyroid, and endocrine organs have been worked too hard and are collapsing. Symptoms that signal low thyroid, like skin and hair changes, fatigue, constipation, and muscle and joint aches, crop up. Cravings for salt, feeling wired but tired, increased light sensitivity, and other adrenal symptoms can manifest. Losing menses can occur, along with acne, worsening PMS symptoms, and polycystic ovarian syndrome (PCOS). All of these are signs of metabolic damage. In other words, the entire nervous system and hormonal system are thrown off, "breaking" the metabolism.
- Meanwhile, in the gastrointestinal system, parasympathetic activity is languishing as a result of chronic stress and stress hormone exposure. Acid production slows, digestive enzymes and juices begin to dry up, cells that line the small intestine are uncoupled, inflammatory processes rev up, and oxidative stress (damage from free radicals) rises. Chronic inflammation and leaky gut translate into malabsorption of amino acids, fatty acids, and nutrients.

⊚ Malabsorption begets mild malnutrition, making it harder for your body
to produce what is needed for digestive fire as well as other crucial factors
for running a healthy body, such as hormones, neurotransmitters, immune
molecules, and antioxidants. No wonder you can't lose weight.

Fixing a broken metabolism requires a little strategy. The nervous system needs
to be rebalanced, concurrently with repairing the gastrointestinal system. As you
begin to soothe your irritated brain and nervous system, your GI system can properly absorb nutrients once again and function fully on all levels. The body finally
starts to manufacture and become sensitive to hormones so that they can do their
job optimally. This will get the scale moving the way you want it to.

Additional Help for Metabolic Damage

Losing weight is not as simple as "eat less and exercise more." There are many
layers and levels of function that stem from the brain and gut in conjunction with
the hormonal system that orchestrate whether you put on weight or burn it off.
Consequently, a multifaceted approach to healing metabolic damage is warranted.
The Gut Restoration Program (page 59) is the place to begin.

Dietary Interventions

With a reduction in cardiovascular exercise, you may need to reduce caloric intake
in order to prevent the weight fluctuations that are so common with this condition. The easiest foods to trim back are calorie-dense items such as nuts, coconut
products, and carbohydrates. Over time, weight fluctuations will stabilize as your
gastrointestinal and hormonal systems normalize.

Lifestyle Interventions

The core issue of metabolic damage stems from an overstimulation of the nervous
system's sympathetic branch and a relative suppression of the parasympathetic
branch. Bringing these two branches into a more functional relationship is crucial
to healing the metabolism. Here are several strategies to help achieve this goal:

Stop jogging. Stop doing excessive cardiovascular exercise. Aerobic exercise
is not inherently bad, of course, but it can aggravate an already overstimulated
nervous system and increases cortisol production.

Replace jogging with outdoor walks. A long, outdoor walk helps to increase the activity of the parasympathetic nervous system and releases feel-good hormones. It also helps burn fat without the dysfunction caused by overexercising.

Replace jogging with weight training. For weight training, it is best to emphasize working on one or two body parts per weight training session, such as chest and back, etc. Choose three to four exercises you like to do, and complete 3–4 sets of each exercise, with ten repetitions per set. Use traditional 3–4 sets of ten with adequate rest in between. Weight training helps balance the nervous system, challenges the heart, and improves blood-sugar control, leading to better body composition (i.e., the amount of lean mass you have in relation to fat mass).

Try restorative yoga, Tai Chi, or Qi-Gong. All of these activities nourish the parasympathetic branch of the nervous system and tell the "fight or flight" response to take a break.

Get into a regular sleep/wake routine. Ditch your night-owl habit, if it is possible. Staying up late stimulates the release of stress hormones that trigger the fight or flight response from your nervous system. Your bedroom should be dark and cool, without electronics and lights beeping and blinking at you. You may even want to consider using a fan or air filter to supply white noise.

Supplements and Herbs

Many supplements can help relink the connection between the brain, nervous system, gastrointestinal system, and hormonal system, helping them to work smoothly and efficiently together to heal a broken metabolism.

Amino acids. Consider amino acids and nutrients that increase GABA production. GABA is the major calming neurotransmitter that helps support the parasympathetic nervous system. A 500 milligram capsule of phenylbutyric acid taken before bed will help increase GABA. Taurine, theanine, vitamin B6, magnesium, zinc, and manganese, taken as a supplement (usually in capsule form), all help the body produce adequate amounts of this feel-good hormone.

Herbs that boost GABA. Valerian root and passionflower are famous for their super-chill effects. In some people, valerian can be stimulating, so just experiment and see what works best for you. Doses for both of these herbs, as a tincture, capsule, or tea, can vary between 100–500 milligrams daily. Start low and go slow.

Herbs that nourish the adrenals. This class of herbs is known as adrenal adaptogens because they help balance adrenal function without overstimulating or suppressing the adrenal glands. Rhodiola is a powerhouse herb in the adaptogenic category. Adaptogens help us "adapt" by not bringing our adrenal adaptogens too high or too low. The dose is 300 milligrams 2–3 times daily. Ashwaganda is another adrenal tonic that is used by some native cultures to increase sexual prowess. Rhodiola and ashwaganda begin to sort out metabolic dysfunction not just by their activity on the adrenal glands but also by buffering the brain against the effects of chronic stress. You can find these tonics in the form of capsules, tinctures, and tea at any natural health food store.

Vitex. If you are having menstrual irregularity, consider taking the herb vitex. Start with 20–80 milligrams daily in capsule form. Vitex can help bring balance to the estrogen/progesterone ratio for women, which can be altered in metabolic damage.

A multivitamin. Consider taking a multivitamin that contains ample B vitamins and at least 5 milligrams of zinc. A consequence of metabolic damage can be mild malabsorption of nutrients, the result of stress-creating imbalances in the GI tract that can lead to inflammation and leaky gut. A multivitamin will help supply nutrients that you may not have been getting from your diet.

Krill oil. Krill oil is rich in phospholipids, a special type of fat that helps repair membranes and improves cellular and nervous system communication. Krill oil (typically supplied in capsules) can help repair the damage wrought by a broken metabolism and supports the nervous, digestive, and hormonal systems. Start with 100 milligrams twice daily.

Ask Your Doctor

Get your vitamin D checked and supplement if your level is below 50. Most labs will say "normal" starts at 30, but there is a big difference between adequate and optimal status. The optimal level is between 50–90. Vitamin D is important for cellular signaling, hormonal balance, and immune function, all of which impact metabolic repair and help you get back on track with weight loss. Take at least 1,000 IU of vitamin D3 per day or more (up to 5,000 IU per day) if you are deficient. You can buy vitamin D3 in gel tabs or drops.

CHAPTER 21

Celiac Disease

Celiac disease is an inherited, autoimmune disease in which the immune system, upon exposure to gluten, attacks and destroys portions of the small intestine. This destruction sets the stage for chronic inflammation, malabsorption, malnutrition, and a cascade of other health consequences, including anemia, infertility, skin rashes, tooth problems, thinning of the bones, and increased likelihood of particular cancers.

The treatment for celiac disease is fairly straightforward—a lifelong avoidance of gluten and gluten-containing products. However, some people who are diagnosed with celiac still don't feel well, even after removing gluten from their diet. In this chapter you'll discover why symptoms persist, how to soothe your entire GI system, and which dietary and lifestyle recommendations will improve your digestive capacity, absorption, and assimilation of foods. If you have been feeling like you need a bit more help and are still having symptoms or issues related to celiac since going gluten-free, this chapter is for you.

Effects of Celiac Disease on Digestion and Beyond

If you have celiac disease and consume gluten, your immune system releases inflammatory molecules that perpetuate an inflammatory response that has local and body-wide effects. Locally, in the small intestine, inflammatory products damage the lining of the gut, blunting the villi (small, fingerlike projections that stick out from the cells that line the small intestine and that absorb nutrition), and create microscopic gaps in the lining of the gut, making it more permeable. Leaky gut quickly becomes established.

On its own, gluten is also able to create gaps in the gut lining, thereby increasing permeability and allowing large molecules, such as partially digested food molecules, pathogens, and environmental toxins, to pass through into the bloodstream. Of course, these large molecules of food or food particles are not supposed to land directly in the bloodstream; they are supposed to be chaperoned through the lining of the small intestine by the cells that line the small intestine. When that wall of cells is breached—as in leaky gut, and as gluten is capable of doing—large molecules can bypass that chaperoning process and drift in. The immune system that is right below the lining now has a way out—through the holes in the leaky gut. So now rogue food particles and the immune system are interacting with each other in a non-chaperoned way. This triggers the immune system to create antibodies that will work against the food particles. If this action goes on long enough, you will develop a sensitivity to a food because when you eat it, your immune system will recognize it as an enemy like it would a virus or harmful bacteria.

As a result, other gastrointestinal symptoms worsen—more bloating, cramping, and gas, along with bowel changes such as increased diarrhea or constipation or a combination of both. Under these circumstances the body is not able to make the full complement of enzymes, acid, bile, and other digestive factors that effectively break down food, and this in turn contributes even more to the body-wide knock-on effects of celiac disease—headache, migraine, fatigue, body aches, joint pain, acne, eczema, rashes, irritability, brain fog, and a host of other symptoms. Because so many symptoms can be caused by celiac, they are often mistaken for something else. Between mounting inflammation and destruction of portions of the gut, dysbiosis of the gut flora also begins to occur. Dysbiosis refers to an imbalance between good, beneficial bacteria and unfavorable or harmful bacteria and yeasts. Fast-growing pathogenic bacteria and yeast are able to compete for space and crowd out normal gut flora.

The effects of celiac disease, as you can see by now, are not simply localized to the digestive system. They have much broader consequences as well, for example in the immune system. IgA is a non-inflammatory immune molecule that is first-line defense against viruses, bacteria, and other pathogens that we may consume or inhale. Typically, IgA levels are low in people who have celiac disease. Consequently, these pathogens are not rendered harmless, and anyone who has celiac is more susceptible to food-borne illness and frequent colds than people who have higher levels of IgA.

The destruction of the lining of the intestine, leaky gut, and increased inflammatory molecules all contribute to the malabsorption of nutrients and malnutrition, which, in turn, is responsible for most of the related conditions and complications of celiac disease, including osteoporosis, anemia, ADHD, infertility, depression, neuropathy, dental-enamel defects, skin conditions, and even certain types of cancer.

The increased inflammatory chemical and immune complexes that circulate throughout the whole body in people who have celiac disease can trigger other autoimmune conditions by "molecular mimicry," when the immune system reacts to and makes antibodies against other tissues in the body because the tissues looks similar from the perspective of the immune system. Autoimmune diseases tends to run in packs, so diabetes type 1, Hashimoto's thyroiditis, autoimmune liver disease, rheumatoid arthritis, lupus, multiple sclerosis, Addison's syndrome, Sjogren's syndrome, Raynaud's syndrome, and complex pain syndromes such as fibromyalgia and chronic fatigue can also be found in those who have celiac disease. For people who have any autoimmune disease, there is a greater likelihood of getting another. Completing the Gut Restoration Program (see page 59) is a way to calm and quell the immune system and restore integrity of the digestive system, hopefully nipping future autoimmune diseases in the bud.

It is safe to say that the vast majority of people who have celiac disease, especially those for whom it has taken years to get a diagnosis, are also looking at the consequences of malnutrition, increased inflammation and dysfunctional immune response, leaky gut, dysbiosis, potential pathogenic infection, and reduced digestive fire.

Why Symptoms Persist

Now that you have an idea how celiac disease creates changes both locally in the small intestine and more broadly in the entire body, you can begin to tease out and understand why some people just don't feel better after cutting out gluten. In a perfect scenario, the intestine would heal itself and begin absorbing food perfectly again; the dysfunctional inflammatory response would cease, gut flora would be restored to normal, enzymatic and acid output would increase, concurrent conditions and symptoms would disappear, and it would all be good. Right?

Right. Yet, this is not the case for some. Too many people still experience symptoms, despite a gluten-free diet. If you are still experiencing symptoms, it is very important to rule out all potential sources of gluten. A common source of the problem, and one that shouldn't be discounted, is gluten that is being consumed unwittingly. To avoid this, read labels on food products very carefully, and check with the manufacturers of medications and cosmetic and household products to make sure they are gluten-free.

If you have been diagnosed with celiac, it could be possible that you also have another autoimmune disease or syndrome that is associated with celiac but which has not yet been diagnosed. Or, you could have an additional gut disorder that mimics the symptoms of celiac, such as microscopic colitis, ulcerative colitis, Crohn's disease, or irritable bowel syndrome (IBS) (although celiac is often misdiagnosed as IBS).

It is far more likely, however, that symptoms of celiac persist because of an underlying digestive problem, rather than any of the scenarios discussed. Low stomach acid, insufficient digestive enzymes and bile, a bacterial or other pathogenic overgrowth, and gut permeability with inflammation will often continue even in the absence of gluten, because these conditions all support and feed off of one another.

Persistent symptoms of celiac may also be attributed to food sensitivities other than gluten. Some of the most common foods to which people develop sensitivity are milk and dairy products, soy, corn, and citrus. These additional sensitivities will continue to drive dysfunctional immune response, leaky gut, and inflammation.

Additional Help for Celiac Disease
The Gut Restoration Program (see page 59) lends itself beautifully to celiac disease because it provides specific nutritional and supplemental support to heal the lining of the small intestine, quell inflammation, boost digestive fire, and balance beneficial bacteria in the gut.

Dietary Interventions
Celiac disease is the clearest example we have today that demonstrates the power of food as medicine. When you remove offending foods—in this case, gluten and

gluten-containing products—and replace them with other foods, you can begin to heal. In addition to swapping out and replacing offending foods, other nutritional strategies can be used to help soothe and nourish the body.

Eat warm, cooked food. If you have been newly diagnosed with celiac disease, it is best to eat most of your food cooked and warm, instead of raw, because it is easily digestible, is soothing, and helps reduce inflammation faster. After you've completed the Gut Restoration Program (see page 59), and your symptoms are stable, you can start to rotate raw food into your diet.

Avoid the trap of gluten-free baked goods. It is easy to feel deprived when you are diagnosed with celiac disease. You may be thinking, "no more pizza, no more bread, no more cookies," and turn to all the gluten-free versions of those foods for comfort. The problem with this strategy is that GF versions are high in refined carbohydrates and low in fiber and protein. They also lack nutrition. A diagnosis of celiac presents you with a unique opportunity to start eating the diet humans were designed to eat: vegetables, fruit, proteins, and healthy fats.

Incorporate coconut products. Coconut is rich in fiber and antimicrobial compounds that help keep pathogenic organisms at bay. In addition, the fatty acids found in coconut provide energy to the cells that line the small intestine and help maintain good gut health.

Have bone broth once a week at the very least. Bone broth contains amino acids, minerals, and collagen-building factors that your body can use to repair the lining of the small intestine. (See recipe for Bone Broth on page 160.) It is one of the best foods you can eat to heal your gut and keep it healthy over the long term.

Lifestyle Interventions

Because the treatment of celiac disease boils down to avoiding gluten for the rest of your life, you will have to make some significant lifestyle adjustments; but if you have celiac, there is no reason to feel overwhelmed or alone. Support for people with this disease is growing by leaps and bounds, and there are plenty of organizations that offer help on how to advocate for yourself and spread awareness.

Find support. Celiac disease is the most common autoimmune disease in the United States, and there are multiple support groups in most regions of the country. Check out Resources (pages 302–303) to find one near you.

Don't be shy about advocating for yourself. Whether you are at a party, dining out at a restaurant, or on the road, you want to be sure that any food you eat is gluten-free.

Read labels on everything. Many products that come into contact with your skin, such as soap, shampoo, conditioner, lotion, makeup, and body wash, contain gluten. Avoid these as well.

Read the labels on your pet's food too. Breathing in the dust from gluten-containing pet kibble is a source of gluten exposure. Luckily, there are many gluten-free and grain-free options available for our furry friends.

Supplements and Herbs

Because one of the major consequences of celiac disease is malabsorption of nutrients, it makes sense to replenish your body with vitamins and minerals in order to compensate for the deficit.

Multivitamin and multi-mineral supplementation. Because malnutrition is a feature of celiac disease, you will have to replenish your stores with non-synthetic, food-based multivitamins and multi-minerals, because they are easier to absorb and tend to be gentler on the system.

Curcumin. A powerful anti-inflammatory herb, curcumin is a known antioxidant that reduces body-wide inflammation and soothes the gut. Take 2 grams, in capsule or powder form, twice daily.

Digestive enzymes and probiotics. Consider long-term supplementation with digestive enzymes and probiotics to help with malabsorption issues, low enzyme and acid output, and lack of digestive fire.

Vitamin D. People with celiac disease typically have very low levels of vitamin D. Take at least 1,000 IU of vitamin D3 daily (capsules, drops, or gel tabs).

Fish oil. Take 3–4 grams of fish oil every day in order to reduce inflammation, improve nerve signaling and conduction, and help heal the lining of the small intestine.

Ask Your Doctor

Celiac is an inherited condition, which means your parents carry the genes and you can pass them to your children, so have everyone in your family tested for celiac.

Consider a bone scan (DEXA scan). Osteoporosis is a major consequence of celiac disease, and a bone scan will let you know if this is something you have to address.

Have your vitamin D, vitamin B12, and folate levels checked. If you have celiac disease, the levels of these nutrients may be low. If your vitamin D level is less than 50, take a supplement, even though 50 is in the "normal" range. Normal does not equal optimal. Optimal levels are between 50 and 90, and if you are not in that range, you may take up to 5,000 IU of vitamin D3 daily. After three months, get your levels rechecked to make sure they are increasing.

Gastrointestinal Health for Kids

Newborn and developing children epitomize both fragility and resiliency. When children are born, the gastrointestinal and related systems are not fully developed. Just as it takes time to reach full adult height, so it takes time for these systems to mature. As children grow and develop, their bodies learn how to deal with a variety of environmental factors—including chemicals and toxins, stress, and of course, food. The first few years of life greatly shape the health of a child, establishing food preferences and susceptibility to eczema, asthma, and environmental and food allergies, and setting the stage for risk of chronic disease later in life.

If a child is stressed, eating inappropriately, or exposed to harmful environmental agents, symptoms can quickly develop in the gastrointestinal tract, immune function, and skin. These factors can also have an effect on behavior. Maybe you've experienced this: Your five-year-old goes to a birthday party; and because it's a special day, you don't see the harm in letting your child have a slice of cake and a cup of soda—foods normally not had at home. Thirty minutes later, your child is running around wildly. Fifteen minutes after that, your child begins to scratch his or her eyes and gets confrontational with the other kids or their parents. An hour or so after cake time, your child is having a tantrum in full meltdown mode.

This example illustrates a one-time event, but what happens to kids when they eat foods that aren't right for their bodies on a more regular basis? As with adults, there has been an enormous rise in the prevalence of gastrointestinal symptoms in children over the last several years. The unique sensitivity of children's bodies, coupled with an ever-harsher environment, means that they may need some extra support. This section explores the underlying causes of gastrointestinal symptoms in the young and what you can do to help your child navigate digestive and digestion-related problems.

The Developing Gastrointestinal System and Gut Restoration

During the first few years of life, a child's gastrointestinal system undergoes radical changes. As organs and systems grow and develop rapidly, these changes can predispose young ones to damage from environmental agents, unhealthy foods, and chronic or excessive stress. In fact, one of the most important strategies for children with chronic gastrointestinal trouble is stress management and reduction. Children are exquisitely sensitive to stress in their environment, and virtually every gastrointestinal complaint in this age group (which includes children up to about age eighteen) can be linked to stress. Luckily, the tremendous energy the body devotes to growth also confers a vitality to children that enables them to heal rapidly and move toward health quickly when given the right input.

How Are Children's Systems Different from Adults'?

Children and adults have the same digestive organs, although the organs of newborn and developing children don't operate at their full adult capacity. Like every other part of their development, the digestive system has to grow and mature.

The digestive system of a newborn baby is set up to handle an easy-to-digest and nutrient-dense source of nourishment: breast milk. Numerous studies have demonstrated that breast milk is the best for babies, in terms of promoting optimal growth and development: higher IQ and lower incidence of allergies, asthma and eczema, and of course, digestive function. Babies are born ready to digest, absorb, and assimilate breast milk, nature's perfect food.

The newness of a baby's gastrointestinal tract does have some unique features that, if given the wrong input, can create gastrointestinal problems or predispose a baby to them later in life. The same can also be said of the immune, skin, hormonal, and neurological systems.

If you were to take a trip down a baby's digestive tract, you would see some notable characteristics of a young and immature system. For starters, the "digestive fire" of a baby is not nearly at the level of an adult's. Digestive fire refers to the production of digestive enzymes—acid and bile—that break down proteins, carbohydrates, and fats into small particles that can readily be absorbed into the system. Nature's solution is to provide a readily digestible and absorbable food source—breast milk. Babies' digestive fire increases as teething approaches and as they get ready to eat solid foods. The stomach and pancreas steadily increase and optimize their production of digestive enzymes and acid, so children are able to progressively digest a wider range of foods.

The small intestine of an infant develops rapidly. The speed of this development, however, makes the small intestine—the major site of action for the absorption of nutrients—more permeable and prone to injury than an adult's. Until the integrity of the small intestine is established, a baby is more vulnerable to common food allergens, such as gluten and dairy, and to gas-causing foods, such as broccoli, cauliflower, and beans, that Mama may be eating. Additionally, harmful environmental agents can have a greater impact on a baby's developing small intestine and pack greater potential for harm.

Moving down from the small intestine to the large intestine, you will note more differences between a baby and an adult. Before birth, a baby's large intestine is not colonized by beneficial bacteria. Babies lack the microbiome—the huge population of friendly bacteria that help us with digestive, metabolic, and immune functions—and must develop it over the first few months and years of life. The first step toward this development is the process of birth itself. Mama's birth canal is rich in friendly, beneficial bacteria, and as a baby is born and moves from the womb to the outside world, bacteria in the vagina inoculates him or her for the first time. Babies delivered by C-section miss this helpful process and, consequently, have higher rates of allergy, asthma, eczema, ear infection, and food sensitivity. Parents can effectively address this lack of inoculation by giving their newborn ⅛–¼ teaspoon of an infant probiotic formula after delivery from a C-section. Breast-feeding mothers can help build their baby's gut flora by supplementing with a daily probiotic or, if the baby is bottle-fed, by adding a pinch of a powdered probiotic to the formula.

Beneficial bacteria help develop the immune system of growing babies. Breast-fed babies have the added benefit and protection of their mother's immune system, which helps shield them from illness via breast milk. As in adults, the majority of a baby's immune system resides in the gastrointestinal tract. The speedily developing immune system of children is not fully online until a child is well past school age—we are all familiar with the frequency of sniffles, colds, and coughs of preschool kids. Young children should recover fairly quickly from this barrage of coughs and sniffles. If your child is not recovering quickly, or if it seems as if he or she is constantly catching colds, getting rashes, or sniffling, it could be that the immune system is struggling because of a gastrointestinal issue. This is most likely because your child is eating a food that causes sensitivity; your child is not properly nourished; or he or she has suboptimal beneficial bacteria that help support the immune system.

Other notable differences between a child's gastrointestinal system and that of an adult's can be seen in the liver. During the first several months and years of a child's life, the liver is quite immature; processes of detoxification, sugar metabolism, and other physiologic functions are rapidly developing. The liver is extra sensitive to environmental inputs such as medications given to the baby or her breast-feeding mother; bisphenol A (BPA), a chemical used in many products, particularly plastics, and known to disrupt hormones; triclosan (an antibacterial and antifungal compound that is in many antibacterial soaps and linked to increased incidence of allergy and antibiotic resistance); pthalates (compounds often added to plastics to soften and increase their flexibility and that are known to disrupt the hormonal system; and parabens (a type of preservative that is added to many soaps, shampoos, lotions, and personal- and body-care products and that are also known to be hormonal/endocrine disruptors). In addition, toys, furniture, and rugs may be off-gassing chemicals, such as volatile organic compounds

(VOCs), that can be deleterious to a baby's developing liver and are best mini-mized if they can't be avoided altogether.

Gut Restoration for Kids

Many of the same elements of gut restoration used for adults, such as finding food sensitivities; supplementing with probiotics, enzymes and other digestive factors; soothing the lining of the digestive tract and healing the intestinal wall; and stress-reduction techniques (see page 95), can be tailored for children. The first step toward reducing symptoms of digestive distress is playing diet detective and ferreting out allergenic foods that the child is eating regularly. Very often, this resolves many issues. Usually, there are one or two food groups—gluten and dairy products top the list—that a child is overconsuming, and as such, the child often doesn't need to do extensive food eliminations that cut out a lot of foods for long periods. With kids, it's very often as simple as that.

You may ask, "Does my child have to avoid this food or that food forever?" and the answer is, "It depends." If a problematic food is creating or worsening your child's complaints, it should be removed from the diet until symptoms resolve. At that time, the food can be reintroduced using the challenge method detailed on page 172. If symptoms return, it is a strong indicator that your child is sensitive to the food and it should be eliminated or challenged, periodically, a few times per year. Some kids outgrow food sensitivities, and some don't.

Dietary supplements

Probiotic supplementation in children is safe and effective at reducing gastroin-testinal symptoms, with the additional benefit of supporting "good" bacteria in the gut. Symptoms such as constipation, diarrhea, eczema, rashes, frequent colds, asthma, and allergies are greatly helped by probiotic supplementation. Probiotics can be used regularly to support optimal health or as needed to manage symp-toms. Although many digestive complaints in children are self-limiting, mean-ing they will eventually resolve, symptoms and distress that have lasted for more than several weeks likely need more support and help. In addition to teasing out food sensitivities and adding probiotics, digestive enzyme supplementation may alleviate symptoms by boosting digestive capacity and the ability to break down proteins, fats, and carbohydrates. A lot of digestive distress, particularly indigestion, gas, and bloating, occurs from this low digestive fire.

A Kid-Friendly Gut Restoration Program

The Gut Restoration Program is easily tailored to children. You will notice that this version is very similar to the adult version (see page 59), with some tweaks specific for young children. The same multifaceted approach of eliminating food sensitivities, supplementing with probiotics, boosting digestive fire, healing and soothing the lining of the gastrointestinal tract, and balancing stress still applies. However, there are a few differences—most of them tailored around the length of time foods are eliminated in order to uncover sensitivities.

Not all kids will need a full Gut Restoration Program. In chapters 23 and 24, common gastrointestinal and gastrointestinal-related conditions are reviewed along with tactics to help children suffering from them. Sometimes these tactics are all that is warranted. If your child is having a hard time resolving symptoms or if the targeted interventions described in chapters 23 and 24 aren't enough, consider initiating the following Gut Restoration Program. Of course, following the program in its entirety, from beginning to end, will not only help resolve symptoms, it will optimize digestive and immune function as well.

1. Remove one to two "big-bully food" items at a time, starting with the foods your child consumes most often (see page 73 for a list of common big-bully foods). The point of this elimination process is to find out which of these commonly allergenic foods are creating or worsening your child's symptoms. If your child has a reaction to a particular food, typically the symptoms will get better in a matter of days after you've removed the offending food for five days. If the symptoms improve, it is likely that your child is sensitive to that food, and it should be greatly minimized, if not completely removed, from your child's diet. If you are not sure if symptoms are improving, reintroduce the food after five days, using the method described on page 172. Watch for symptoms to flare up when the food is reintroduced. If they flare, that food is

a culprit and should be eliminated for another four weeks. You can then try to reintroduce the food once again. If your child reacts with symptoms, that food should be eliminated over the long term.

Breast-feeding mothers can follow the same protocol for themselves, eliminating one to two foods at a time from their diet and watching symptoms in their baby. Breast-feeding mothers may choose to consider eliminating foods from the cruciferous family of vegetables—for example, broccoli, kale, cauliflower, bok choi, cabbage, and Brussels sprouts—along with onions, garlic, caffeine, and eggs.

2. Give your child ⅛ teaspoon or ¼ teaspoon of probiotic powder daily, depending on his or her age. See page 84 to find out how to choose a probiotic.

3. Give your child one pinch of digestive enzyme powder with each meal, if your child is younger than five years old. Use a larger dose—⅛ teaspoon—for kids over the age of five. Most digestive enzymes are sold in capsule form. Open the capsule and mix a pinch or so in with food. Enzymes can easily be mashed into veggies, scrambled with eggs, and mixed into drinks or just about anything. Enzymes help break down food, ease digestion, and reduce gas and bloating.

4. Give your child 1.5 grams of glutamine powder twice daily if your child is over four years old. Glutamine mixes easily into water and has a mild, if somewhat chalky, taste. Glutamine is a powerful agent that helps heal and soothe the lining of the gastrointestinal tract.

5. Try the stress management techniques on page 190.

Follow steps 1 through 5 for four weeks and then evaluate your child's symptoms. If your child is feeling 75 percent or more better, discontinue glutamine (see step 4) and halve the amount of probiotics and enzymes (see steps 2 and 3) for two weeks, and then discontinue probiotics and enzymes. If your child is not showing 75 percent improvement, he or she should stay on the program (steps 1 through 5) for another two to four weeks, and then reevaluate the symptoms.

A Deeper Look at Symptoms

The Gut Restoration Program is a simple way to greatly improve digestive and digestion-related issues in infants and children. If symptoms are not improving, there may be a hidden cause that is still driving them—an undiscovered food sensitivity, for example—in which case, testing is an option. Look for a health-care provider who can give your child an IgG food-sensitivity test. If you cannot find a provider to do an IgG test, there are companies online that can help you (see Resources on page 303 for a list). Bacterial dysbiosis—an imbalance between good, beneficial bacteria and harmful, pathogenic bacteria or yeast—can also be responsible for unresolved symptoms. Children with a history of antibiotic use and a low-fiber, high-sugar diet are more at risk for bacterial dysbiosis. Parasitic infection is another common reason for unremitting symptoms, most particularly symptoms that are cyclical. Although we don't like to think about it very much, it is exceedingly easy to pick up a parasite. They are found not only in tropical or developing countries, but can also be picked up from other children, day care, restaurants, pets, or just from playing outside. The best tool to evaluate dysbiosis, yeast overgrowth, parasitic infection, and digestive function is a comprehensive digestive stool analysis (CDSA). This stool test quantifies the amount of beneficial bacteria in the gut as well as the number of bad guys that could be creating problems. Additionally, a CDSA can help uncover inflammation in the digestive system and give an idea of the digestive ability and absorptive capacity of the child. This test, as its name implies, is extremely comprehensive, and pinpoints undiscovered reasons for gastrointestinal distress in both adults and children. CDSA tests are noninvasive and yield an enormous amount of useful information. Some insurance covers these tests as well. For more information about CDSA, see page 218.

Common Childhood Conditions

In this chapter, you'll learn more about the most common conditions found in infancy and childhood and learn practical solutions that can help your child feel better. From constipation and colic to skin conditions and asthma, there is a lot that can be done to support the health of your little ones. Note that the condition-specific interventions discussed in this chapter can be used by themselves or in conjunction with the children's version of the Gut Restoration Program (see page 263). Also remember that, for all of their fragility, infants and children are wonderfully resilient and their bodies will bounce back to health when they are given the right support.

Colic, Reflux, and Silent Reflux

These three conditions contain a constellation of overlapping symptoms that represent perhaps the most common that occur during infancy. The symptoms of colic, which include gassiness and inconsolable crying for several hours—usually around the same time of day—should be carefully differentiated from reflux and silent reflux. Reflux can share symptoms of colic, accompanied by spitting up, often after feeding, and sometimes projectile vomiting, tightness in the abdomen, fussiness, and crying. Silent reflux is termed silent because there may be no obvious signs of reflux, such as vomiting, so symptoms masquerade as colic. Babies who are congested, snuffling, and snoring, catch colds regularly, or seem like they frequently have a cold, may have silent reflux—a misnomer because babies who have this condition are anything but silent.

Causes

Colic and reflux stem from the same root causes:

◎ **Diet.** To uncover the causes of reflux, it is important to find out exactly which foods are being eaten by both the mother and her baby. In babies who are formula fed, look to the ingredients in the formula as a potential cause of reflux. In babies who are breast-fed, look to the mother's diet for the cause. The most common foods that cause or worsen colic and reflux in babies also tend to be milk and gluten products, because they are the easiest and most filling foods for new moms to eat with one hand and on the run! Other foods in Mom's diet, such as onions, garlic, and cruciferous veggies such as broccoli, cabbage, cauliflower, kale, bok choi, and Brussels sprouts, can also create or worsen colic.

◎ **Nervous system.** Studies show that women who have had stressful pregnancies are more likely to have babies with colic. This has to do with the overstimulation of the sympathetic branch of the nervous system—the fight or flight branch—which, when overstimulated, dominates (and renders less functional) the rest and digest branch of the nervous system. The end result is higher stress, worse digestive function, and greater likelihood that their babies will have colic.

  The birth experience can also cause tummy troubles for a baby later on. Birth trauma and complicated birth can stimulate the fight or flight branch of the nervous system, making colic and reflux more likely to develop. The first few days and weeks of life are stressful for new babies as they make the dramatic adjustment from the familiar environment of the womb to the bright, stimulating world into which they have been abruptly delivered. Is it any surprise that their digestive systems need some time to catch up with this enormous change? In addition, the environment and stress levels at home for new parents can have a significant impact on newborns. Anxiety, depression, and lack of resources and support are overwhelmingly common in the parents of babies with reflux.

◎ **Medications.** Antibiotics are always prescribed as a pretreatment for women who are undergoing a C-section and are often prescribed in routine hospital births, particularly for women who are positive for the bacteria group

B Streptococcus. Babies who are transferred to the neonatal intensive care unit (NICU) are often admitted for respiratory conditions and are given antibiotics there. This use of antibiotics at or around birth makes it more likely that reflux and/or colic will develop—not to mention that early antibiotic use can harm the burgeoning population of beneficial bacteria that colonize the large intestine.

Additional Help for Reflux and Colic

Now that we've explored the most common causes for reflux—diet, stress, and medication—we can begin to do something about it. The following are tried-and-true tips and tricks to reduce the symptoms of colic, reflux, and silent reflux. The best way to approach the vulnerable and developing system of a young infant is to consider all of the factors that may have caused colic and reflux to develop in the first place. By addressing diet, the nervous system, and other factors, while managing symptoms, your baby will be happier—and so will you!

Symptoms of colic and reflux tend to resolve by the time a baby is four to six months old, even without treatment. In the event that treatment is initiated, it is common to see a 30 percent reduction in symptoms in one week to ten days. By the time three to four weeks have passed, babies should be feeling 50–75 percent better, which will be evidenced by a reduction in symptoms. All interventions, including drug therapy with acid-blocking drugs, take time to work and reduce symptoms. It is important for your sanity, as a parent, to be aware of the timetable associated with treatment and know what to expect and when to expect it.

Nutrition

Breast-fed babies often find it difficult to digest the same foods that give their mothers digestive troubles. It may take a little detective work to find out which foods are giving a baby digestive distress. Some of the common offenders (for both mothers and their babies) are gluten, dairy, soy, fatty foods, gassy veggies such as broccoli, cauliflower, cabbage, kale, bok choi and brussels sprouts, onions, garlic, beans and legumes, spicy foods, and caffeine.

To find out more about a nursing baby's food sensitivities, try taking these steps:

- If you're a nursing mother, eliminate one food at a time for three to five days, starting with the most likely culprit. Often, it is the food you are consuming the most of, a food that is a classic "colic culprit," such as gassy veggies, or the food you suspect is most problematic for you. It is important to find substitutions for the food you are eliminating, in order to make the trial as stress-free as possible. During the elimination period, watch the baby's symptoms. If they improve by one-fourth or more, it is likely that the suspect food is in fact a contributing factor to reflux and colic.

- After three to five days, have one to two servings of the "trial" food and watch the baby's symptoms. If they flare, your baby is reacting to that food and you should avoid it for the duration of breast-feeding. Of course, you do not have to reintroduce a food that you know your baby reacts to—reintroductions should be made when you can't quite tell if the elimination of a food has helped improve symptoms.

- Eliminate the next suspect on your list. It is not necessary to eliminate multiple foods at a time in order to determine your baby's (and potentially your) sensitivity to them. Taking out too many foods at once is stressful, and it can feel particularly restrictive to nursing moms who need dense nutrition. Playing the one-food-at-a-time detective is just fine.

- As a breast-feeding mom, there are a few foods and herbs that you can actually add to your daily or weekly nutrition to help soothe your baby's colic. For example, fennel root, when it is sliced or shredded into a salad or eaten plain, is an anti-gas herb that has been used for generations as one of the main ingredients in "gripe water," a home remedy for infants with colic, reflux, and other stomach ailments. Ginger, taken as a fresh or dried tea or used as an ingredient in cooking, goes a long way toward reducing gas associated with colic. Chamomile is another herb that decreases gas and spasm and is quite lovely and easy to take in tea form.

- Mint tea should be avoided by women who are breast-feeding colicky babies and babies with reflux, because mint can dilate the lower esophageal sphincter (LES), creating a path for stomach contents to splash up into the esophagus.

- If you are giving your baby formula, consider using a hypoallergenic product. Earth's Best Organic Infant Formula, for example, is easily obtainable in grocery stores and can be easy for babies to digest.

How to De-stress Your Baby

Too often, parents are simply handed a prescription for their baby and sent on their way without further information or a time line of when to expect an improvement in their baby's symptoms. It is completely normal for parents to have increased stress with a colicky baby and emotional support is crucial from friends, family, and medical-care providers. By arming parents with information and a time line, it is possible to reduce stress in the entire household.

Babies' little bodies go through a lot during birth, and although they are wonderfully flexible and moldable, sometimes they can experience minor structural changes in the skull, muscles, or skeletal structure that can impact the nervous system and warrant hands-on medicine. Two examples are craniosacral therapy, the gentle alignment of the skull and spine, and chiropractic medicine, which adjust and optimizes the skeletal structure. Both therapies address and soothe the nervous system via the musculoskeletal system. A course of treatment over several weeks by a craniosacral therapist or a chiropractor can be very helpful in de-stressing your baby.

Probiotic Support

Supplemental probiotics restore gut bacteria and help babies assimilate nutrients and are particularly helpful for babies who are formula fed and are not getting beneficial bacteria through their mother's milk. Find a powdered product that contains *Bifidus rhamnosus* and *B. infantis*. The dose is ⅛ teaspoon twice daily, mixed into a bottle of breast milk or formula or mixed on a spoon with several drops of breast milk or formula and tipped into the baby's mouth. Klaire Labs makes a wonderful infant probiotic. Jarrow's Baby's Jaro-Dophilus and Pharmax HLC Neonate also have infant formulas, but note that both of these contain dairy and should not be given to little ones who are sensitive to dairy products.

Herbal Remedies

Gripe water. Perhaps one of the easiest herbal remedies to obtain—and the most effective anti-gas treatment for colic—is gripe water, a liquid combination of several herbs including chamomile, fennel, and ginger. Administered in a dropper, gripe water helps dissolve gas and reduce associated discomfort. The dose is 10 drops with feedings, given in a bottle or placed on a spoon and given directly to your baby. It is important to be consistent about using gripe water regularly, if your baby has colic, so that it can start dissolving gas and reducing painful spasms before symptoms kick in. You can find gripe water at your local pharmacy or health food store.

Herbal teas. An alternative to gripe water is a brew made from one bag of chamomile tea and one bag of fennel tea. Put the tea bags into a mug and pour hot water over them. Let the tea bags steep for 5–7 minutes, and then let the tea cool. The dose is ½ teaspoon at every feeding.

Deglycyrrhizinated licorice (DGL). DGL helps soothe inflammation in the esophagus and lining of the stomach. For babies with silent or projectile reflux, add DGL to breast milk or formula. Scientific Botanicals, Inc. makes a powdered form of DGL, or you can buy chewable DGL wafers from a pharmacy or health food store and crush them with the back of a spoon. The dose is ¼ teaspoon three times daily, with meals.

Digestive enzymes. For tough cases of colic and reflux, digestive enzymes can be used. Combine ¼ teaspoon DGL, ⅛ teaspoon probiotics, a pinch of digestive enzymes, and enough breast milk to create a smooth paste, and pop it into your baby's mouth twice daily.

Medication
Sometimes a medication such as baby Zantac or Prevacid has to be used for symptoms of reflux or colic. Typically, these drugs are used only for a few weeks to months. It is completely safe and helpful to use any of the measures discussed—herbal remedies, probiotics, etc.—in conjunction with medication. Keep in mind, however, that these drugs fundamentally block stomach-acid production, making it harder for babies to digest food. There are two major consequences of medicating reflux with acid blockers that have been observed clinically: 1) the onset of constipation with the introduction of solid food and 2) feeding problems due to lowered motility and function of the gastrointestinal system.

Constipation
For toddlers and school-aged kids, constipation tops the list of the most common conditions. The causes of constipation vary according to age, diet, stressors, and

exposure to pathogens. The role diet plays in toddlers who are constipated is undeniable: nutrition is overwhelmingly responsible for bowel function in kids, just as it is for adults, but other factors can come into play as well. For example, power struggles that crop up around food can arise during the toddler phase and cause constipation. Kids who aren't introduced to and don't eat a wide variety of foods and who nosh primarily on gluten and dairy products are also more likely to be constipated. In addition, there is a cultural bias in the United States that puts pressure on parents to give milk to their children. The irony is that milk is the food most likely to constipate young ones. Resolution of constipation is possible with a few key targeted interventions, such as dietary changes and behavior modifications.

Cow's Milk

Cow's milk is certainly not the only way to get calcium from food. In fact, kale, collard greens, turnip greens, almonds, parsley, watercress, dried figs, and sunflower seeds have more calcium per ounce than cow's milk. Buckwheat, sesame seeds, olives, broccoli, walnuts, pecans, miso, apricots, raisins, dates, artichokes, cabbage, cashews, sweet potato, and brown rice also contain calcium. Cow's milk is a common food allergen and a major driver of constipation in kids. Interestingly, many children who have an allergy to gluten will also have a concurrent sensitivity to milk products. There are a couple reasons why this may be so. The protein molecules in both gluten and dairy products are highly inflammatory and allergenic and can create similar responses from the immune system. Lactose intolerance—an inability to digest milk sugar—is documented alongside cases of celiac disease—the autoimmune genetic condition of gluten intolerance. Lastly, it is well known that gluten molecules pass through human breast milk, and there is no reason to think that the same isn't true of cow's milk. Cows that are fed gluten-containing grains are going to have gluten residues in their milk, which can trigger a response in gluten-sensitive kids. If you suspect this may be the case for your child, you can experiment with grass-fed milk and milk products to see if your baby reacts to them the way he or she does to non-grass-fed milk (most conventional milk, by the way, including organic milk, is not grass-fed). Give your child two servings of grass-fed milk for one day only and assess his symptoms over three days. If your child's symptoms do not worsen, it could be that grass-fed milk can be tolerated and previous symptoms were a reaction to gluten in conventional milk.

Causes

Most toddlers in day care aren't getting enough veggies and fiber because they aren't given a variety of healthy choices for snacks and meals. Instead, standard day-care fare usually consists of cream cheese, Goldfish, fruit, and milk—a perfect storm for constipation. Indeed, a high-dairy, high-sugar, low-fiber diet tops the list for the most common reason kids are constipated. There are a number of other factors that can contribute to constipation as well:

- **Lack of sleep.** Without enough sleep, lots of kids literally run on adrenaline—an increased fight or flight response that slows bowel motility. While every child is different, it is generally recommended that two-year-olds get between 10 and 13 hours of sleep a night. Three-year-olds can handle a little less sleep but still need naps or periods of quiet downtime with low stimulation. A generation ago, children in kindergarten took naps every day, which is not so true anymore. Lack of regular sleep contributes to increased stress and decreased bowel motility (i.e., the bowel is slowed down; regular bowel movements don't occur, and constipation is the result).
- **Inactivity.** Physical activity stimulates the digestive system and acts like an abdominal massage to get things going. Exercise helps stimulate the enteric nervous system of the gut—the "brain" of the digestive tract that helps regulate bowel movements—and the digestive organs and intestines themselves, which greatly helps with bowel regularity. Lack of movement does the reverse.
- **Forced potty training.** Trying to potty train a child who is not ready or using negative punishment methods while potty training ensures that a child will never want to have a bowel movement. Potty training should be as stress free as possible, with the focus on neutral or positive reinforcement.
- **Medications.** Current or prior use of acid-blocking drugs such Zantac and Prevacid can disrupt peristalsis (the rhythmic, pulsing movement of the

intestines that pushes food down and out of the digestive tract) and cause constipation. Antibiotics, typically given to toddlers and young kids for ear infections, alter the balance of beneficial gut flora, which in turn impairs gut function and can cause constipation.

Additional Help for Constipation in Toddlers

Although constipation is troubling and can sometimes be a devastating problem, it can be remedied fairly easily with the right approach. Taking an honest look at your child's nutrition, water intake, activity levels, and sleep will help you resolve the issue. Additionally, there are several readily available supplements that can aid in relieving constipation. If symptoms don't improve with the following interventions, consider initiating the Kid-Friendly Gut Restoration Program on page 263.

Nutrition

Doctors agree that healthy nutrition is the most important issue to address in constipation. Adjusting the way kids eat ultimately means working with the way the whole family eats. If a child's family doesn't eat in a healthy, balanced way, the child is not going to eat well either. Lack of fiber and an imbalanced diet are a surefire way to induce constipation.

The majority of the diet for toddlers and kids should consist of proteins and fresh vegetables and fruits—not grain and dairy products. You can add variety to your child's diet by changing things up a little, i.e., providing different kinds of things to eat at snack time, rather than relying on the same one or two snacks every day.

Dehydration, along with lack of fiber, is another major factor in the development of constipation. The right type of fluid is key. Milk is inherently constipating, and juice, which is packed with sugar, can also negatively impact gut motility. To address these issues, simply dilute your child's milk and juice with water. Often, this process is more about weaning the parent than the toddler! Parents ultimately make the decision about what their children eat and drink, and when they report that "it's hard" to make the swap to water, parents are usually referring to the discomfort of watching their child have a tantrum. Once this storm is weathered, however, most kids are content to drink water. To ease the adjustment you can start gradually, by watering down juice and milk a little bit at a time.

Healthy fats are a cornerstone of healthy digestion and, along with fiber and water, help ease the transit of food through the digestive tract. Healthy fats act as a lubricant, easing the passage of stool. Fatty acids—including any of these healthy fats—can be used in conjunction with one another to improve bowel function:

- **Fish or cod liver oil.** Supplementation of 1 gram of combined EPA and DHA from fish or cod liver oil will help greatly with constipation. Several flavored, kid-friendly versions are available, including a delicious product called Barlean's Omega Swirl that works well for kids who have a picky palate.

- **Ground flaxseed/flax oil.** The beneficial fats in flax are a good alternative to fish oils for children who won't take fish oil or who are vegetarian or vegan. One to two tablespoons of ground flaxseed can easily be added to your child's diet, but be sure that he increases his daily water intake by 8 ounces or so, because ground flaxseed also contains fiber. If it is added to a dehydrated system, the fiber can make symptoms of constipation worse or cause symptoms of gas and bloating. A good rule of thumb is to always increase water whenever you add extra fiber to the diet, whether it's yours or your children's! Alternatively, you can give your child a dose of 1–2 teaspoons of flax oil daily. Note that some children are irritated by flax, so you should monitor symptoms after you've given your child flaxseed or flax oil.

- **Coconut oil and coconut products.** Another option for a healthy, beneficial fat is coconut oil and/or coconut butter and other coconut products, such as shredded coconut, coconut milk, and coconut flour. Kids can have 2 teaspoons to 1 tablespoon of any one of these every day to help with constipation. Coconut oil can be drizzled over veggies, mixed into a smoothie, or used to cook eggs or meats. Coconut butter is delicious off the spoon or spread on apples, carrots, and celery. Coconut milk can be used in soups, stews, and smoothies or taken with a pinch of cinnamon. In addition, coconut fat helps lubricate the digestive system and makes bowel movements easier. Coconut has many gut-boosting components such as medium-chain triglycerides that act as a source of energy for the digestive system and also have mild antimicrobial properties that help keep bad guys at bay.

- **Probiotic supplementation.** Probiotics promote regularity, help boost immune function, and reduce the incidence of ear infections, allergies, asthma, and eczema. Powdered forms of probiotics are readily available and are easy for kids to take because they can be mixed into drinks or food or can simply be poured onto the tongue. The dose is ¼ teaspoon twice daily, taken with food. (See page 84 for more details about probiotic supplements.)

◉ **Enzyme tablets.** Chewable, flavored, digestive enzyme tablets work wonders for toddlers. One-half of a tablet taken two to three times daily between meals helps improve bowel function. Start with one-half tab twice daily and work up to half a tablet three times daily over the course of several days.

◉ **Magnesium supplements.** Magnesium helps relax the digestive system, aiding in regularity—a great help to kids and people of any age, for that matter, who have constipation. Magnesium is inexpensive and readily available in drug and health food stores alike. Try 200 milligrams of magnesium glycinate before bed. The dose of magnesium can be worked up slowly over the course of several days. Too much magnesium will result in loose stools, so watch carefully. If your child develops loose stools or diarrhea, reduce the dose.

Additional Help for Constipated School-Aged Kids (Older than Five Years)

Keep talking with your kids. After potty training, parents should continue to follow up with their children about their bathroom habits. Issues related to constipation and stomach pain can crop up after potty training simply because they have not been addressed. It's helpful to talk to your kids about what is considered normal bowel function. While there are various opinions about what is considered normal among children in the five- to eighteen-year-old range, most experts agree that kids should move their bowels once to twice daily. This is a sign that they are eating enough food and fiber. The stool should be well formed and easy to pass. It should not be pale and float on top of the water; neither should it look like rabbit pellets. The volume of stool per day should be the equivalent of about two handfuls (your child's, that is).

Rest and sleep are critical. School-aged kids face a real schedule change when they head off to school. Often, sleep is inadequate because they are staying up later at night and getting up earlier in the morning. Children's days are often so heavily scheduled with studies, practice of one kind or another, and events that they have little to no downtime or rest during the day. In addition, some kids can be a little shy about having a bowel movement in a public place and may have difficulties even discussing the issue, so try to be gentle and matter-of-fact when bringing it up.

Dealing with the School Day

A typical school day is about 7 hours long. Most kids have something to eat and drink only at lunch, which means they may not be getting enough to eat and drink to sustain them healthily over the course of the school day. Combining lack of sleep with an environment in which kids are overworked, overcommitted, under-rested, malnourished, and thirsty elevates stress hormones and puts kids in a stressful state that doesn't support great digestive function or bowel regularity. Consequently, gastrointestinal issues can manifest or worsen, and behavioral issues, such as defiance, lashing out, misbehaving, acting inappropriately, etc., sometimes arise. Unfortunately, a child may know that he or she feels "off" but may not question that feeling if the child has never felt any other way. That's why it's so important to keep talking to your kids (without being obsessive) about how they're feeling and asking how often they're having regular bowel movements.

Honoring Your Children's Need for Downtime and Rest

Sadly, American culture promotes overwork in the name of education and values it as a marker of success and good parenting. Parents innocently and inadvertently put their wishes for what they think is best for their children ahead of what is actually best for them. Time for sleep, rest, and mealtime with the family should be fiercely protected, even if it means scheduling fewer events or commitments for your child.

Ask Your Doctor

Constipated children who also have other conditions such as eczema, ear infections, seasonal allergies, and frequent colds most likely have at least one food or environmental sensitivity (if not more) and should be tested for them.

Eczema and Atopic Dermatitis

While it may not seem immediately intuitive that a skin condition like eczema is also a gastrointestinal issue, the two are intimately connected. During pregnancy, the gastrointestinal system and skin are developing at the same time, from the same cells. The skin often acts as a mirror for what is going on inside the gastrointestinal system because of this relationship. As children grow rapidly, and as their gastrointestinal and immune systems mature, skin disturbances commonly appear. Typically, these are short-lived and go away on their own, but sometimes a more chronic condition, such as eczema or atopic dermatitis, can develop. Dryness and flaking of the skin, redness, itching, and sometimes oozing and crusting of the skin are common in eczema and atopic dermatitis. It can be found anywhere on the body, but is common behind the ears, at the base of the skull, on the scalp, behind the knees, and in the creases of the elbows.

Infants and children who develop eczema are also more likely to have environmental and food allergies and may have a higher disposition toward asthma. This triad of conditions is referred to as **atopy** and can be influenced by a number of factors, including food and environmental allergy, the balance of beneficial bacteria, environmental pollution, stress, and even the weather.

Healing the Skin

Because the skin and gastrointestinal and immune systems are linked, integrative and complementary health providers often treat and support the gastrointestinal system—and in turn the immune system—in order to heal the skin. In turn, identifying food sensitivities, supplementing with probiotics and skin-supporting fatty acids, and soothing and healing the gastrointestinal lining will also support and heal the skin and alleviate symptoms of eczema, dermatitis, and other skin conditions. Up to 15 percent of all infants experience eczema or atopic dermatitis, so it's important to have some tools to help alleviate the symptoms of eczema. Try these strategies:

⊚ **Find and minimize exposure to environmental allergens: dust, dust mites, trees, pollen, animals and their dander.** Smoke and synthetic fragrances are common inhalant (breathed-in) allergens. Allergens such as soaps, shampoo, lotions, laundry and dish detergent, and metals (particularly nickel) can also trigger a response when they come into contact with the skin.

- **Consider IgE food-allergy testing.** This skin-prick test will uncover fast-acting food allergies. Many people with eczema have IgE food allergies, and some studies suggest 60–80 percent of kids have an IgE allergy to at least one food.
- **Consider IgG food-allergy testing.** IgG food sensitivities are responsible for slower, more chronic symptoms that can extend to the skin. It is common for both kids and adults to have IgG food sensitivities if they also have eczema.
- Rule out dysbiosis (an imbalance of good and bad bacteria in the large intestine) and yeast overgrowth with a comprehensive digestive stool analysis (CDSA). See page 218 for more information on the CDSA.
- Use hypoallergenic and natural household cleaning and hygienic products, and make sure that your child uses hypoallergenic soaps, shampoos, lotions, and toiletries because many products contain additives compounds and harsh chemicals that irritate skin.
- Supplement your child's diet with probiotics. In numerous studies, use of probiotics has been shown to reduce the severity and frequency of eczema. Probiotics help keep beneficial gut flora happy and balance the immune system. Women who are breast-feeding should take 50 billion CFUs daily of a soy- and dairy-free hypoallergenic formula. Infants and kids who are no longer breast-feeding should take ⅛–¼ teaspoon of a powdered probiotic daily.
- Breast-feed for at least six months or longer if you can. Babies who are breast-fed have less eczema as well as a lower incidence of asthma, ear infections, allergies, and missed days of school.

Additional Help for Eczema & Atopic Dermatitis

Other strategies to help alleviate the symptoms of eczema and atopic dermatitis include the use of oils, creams, and salves, along with proper hydration and plenty of vitamin C–rich foods (or supplements):

Topical coconut oil. This oil softens and strengthens the skin and has a long history of use. It is extremely safe and free of additives, synthetic compounds, parabens, pthalates, fragrances, and preservatives—the junk found in many lotions and skin-care products. Coconut oil has antiseptic and antifungal properties too. It does not have side effects, unlike steroids that are often used for eczema and that thin the skin, making it more susceptible to damage, injury, and infection. Topical coconut oil also works extremely well in cases of cradle cap.

Creams or salves that contain calendula, chamomile, licorice, chickweed, or a combination of these herbs. Modern scientific literature has shown that all of these herbs that have been used traditionally to heal the skin can hold their own against hydrocortisone creams—and without any of the negative side effects.

Fermented cod liver oil (FCLO). Although there really isn't much research to support its use (compared to unfermented fish oils), FCLO seems to be quite effective for treating eczema, but because it is fermented, FCLO tastes pretty funky compared to regular cod liver oil, flax oil, or coconut oil. The dose is 1–2 tablespoons taken daily. It is the rare toddler who will happily gulp this down. Try hiding fermented cod liver oil in a smoothie or in veggies.

Other beneficial fats. Incorporating healthy fats into the diet, such as coconut oil, ground flaxseeds, flax oil, and evening primrose oil, can help alleviate eczema. Studies show that people with eczema have lower levels of healthy fatty acids than those who do not.

Adequate hydration. Mild dehydration is not good for the skin. One of the jobs of the skin is to trap and hold moisture. When your child isn't getting enough water, skin is more likely to be dry. A good rule of thumb for water intake for kids is to take their weight in pounds and divide by two. This number is the amount of water in ounces your child should be drinking daily, with a bit more added in for high-activity children. (For example, a 50-pound child should drink about 25 ounces of water a day: $50 \div 2 = 25$.)

Increase vitamin C–rich foods or consider supplementation. Small studies have shown that vitamin C can help alleviate symptoms of eczema. Vitamin C is a building block of collagen, so it makes sense that by boosting collagen production you can heal the skin. Low-allergen foods that are rich in vitamin C are berries, leafy greens, apricots, sweet potatoes, and kiwis. You could also consider supplementing your child with 200–500 milligrams of vitamin C daily in the form of Ester-C.

CHAPTER 24

Building a Healthy Digestive System

Parents want their children to thrive, but raising kids in today's complex, challenging world can be tough. Putting energy toward creating a more secure, balanced, and peaceful environment for your young ones will help them develop strong and healthy bodies, inside and out. In this chapter, you will find out how to best support your growing children, using common-sense nutrition and other lifestyle tips, and how to protect them against harmful environmental agents (including cleaning and personal-care products), foods, and excessive stress. While these factors may not be the only culprits, they're certainly a part of the big picture. By learning about your child's unique sensitivities and coping styles, you can best use the tools here to provide the best environment for them to grow and thrive.

A Formula for Digestive Success

In today's world, we live with an ever-increasing number of pollutants, chemicals, toxins, pesticides, herbicides, heavy metals, electromagnetic pollution, noise pollution, light pollution, and a variety of other assaults. The combination of air, soil, and water pollution put extra stress on young children's developing systems, making them more prone to a host of digestive and immune complaints and symptoms. If you layer into this equation the wide availability of cheap, nutritionally devoid, addictive foods (that high-paid marketing professionals have convinced your children to eat), you have the perfect environment for sickness to develop. However, it doesn't have to be this way. Reducing your child's exposure to environmental toxins, stress, and noise from an increasingly loud, electronic world and ensuring that he or she eats a balanced diet is a powerful means of supporting the health of your child's digestive system—a campaign that entails just a few steps that any parent can master.

Keep It Clean . . . Lick the Chlorine

A recent study linked exposure to chlorine with food allergies, a threat that can easily be addressed with a water filtration system, especially as inexpensive and easy-to-install models are readily available. Chlorine also disrupts the hormonal system and has been shown to harm the beneficial bacteria that live in the gut and that provide innumerable helpful functions, including aiding in digestion, nutrient absorption and assimilation, and immune system function. These beneficial bacteria even help reduce the risk of cardiovascular disease and keep us trim. What's more, the benefits of clean water extend far beyond reducing risk for food sensitivity. Water is another point of entry for countless compounds, such as pharmaceutical drugs, metals, fluoride, and other compounds that can wreak havoc with our health—all the more reason to filter the water your family uses! Another way to reduce exposure to toxic compounds is to use natural or organic cleaning, household, and personal-care products.

Stay Calm

When the body is under stress, regardless of where the stress is coming from, the sympathetic branch of the nervous system, also known as the fight or flight branch, becomes dominant. This response is all very well and good if you actually have to run away from or quickly deal with a threatening situation, but if the fight or flight response becomes the body's preferred means of dealing with stress, serious digestive problems can crop up. This occurs when the other branch of the nervous system—the parasympathetic branch, also known as the rest and digest branch—takes a back seat to the fight or flight branch. The rest and digest branch promotes optimal production of enzymes, acid, and other digestive factors that help the stomach stay calm and relaxed, while promoting normal, regular movement of the gastrointestinal tract. When these functions are suppressed by high-stress digestive disturbances, indigestion, reflux, stomach pains, constipation, diarrhea, and the like can emerge. Chronic stress can also negatively impact sleep and school performance.

Although every child is different, there are a few strategies you can use to help reduce stress and thus support your child's rest and digest branch—and healthy digestion. Children want to know that they are loved and accepted no matter what, and it is important, as a parent, that you reassure them of that on a regular basis. Learn what your children's triggers are for stress or anxiety and help them to understand what the triggers are. Strategize with them about ways that they can make those experiences less stressful. Next, make sure that your children have enough downtime throughout the day—at least 2 hours' worth of unscheduled time—when they can relax. Keeping a consistent bedtime routine helps to ensure enough sleep for your children and prevents potentially stressful disruptions in that routine. Taking a walk together after school or dinner will also help lower stress hormones and build wonderful connections that are stress reducing all on their own.

Try some of these methods to help ensure a calm, relaxing, and supportive environment for your child's digestive health and general well-being:

- **Stay in touch, literally.** Babies and toddlers love to be touched. It's also a great way to bond with your child. A gentle massage, whether it is full body or just the belly, legs, and feet, calms the nervous system and may even promote better sleep. It certainly is a good way to help your child feel relaxed. Use coconut oil and a few drops of lavender oil to gently massage your toddler for a particularly delicious and relaxing experience.
- **Make your home a haven.** Although it is not always possible to keep things mellow and quiet, it is still a good idea to maintain home as a place of rest and sanctuary instead of a place of stress and chaos. Consider keeping electronics out of your children's bedrooms and turn them off in other places in the house when they are not actually being used.
- **Establish a good sleep routine** with a regular bedtime and pre-bedtime activities, like a soothing bath and story time, as opposed to a mad dash to get to bed.
- If you are open to it, and your child is old enough, **teach him or her about meditation** and staying in the moment. This could be as simple as asking your child to periodically notice his or her thoughts. Deep breathing is a technique that is easily learned and something kids can do anywhere. Teach your child to breathe deeply into the belly, filling the lungs with air, whenever tension is felt.

◉ **Balance the whole family's diet.** Quite often, gastrointestinal symptoms are the result of imbalanced eating. The overconsumption of certain foods such as milk and grain products, coupled with low intake of fibrous veggies, is at the root of the problem. In fact, most American children don't eat the recommended number of vegetables that they should eat in order to stay healthy. Part of the problem is our own poor modeling as parents. Our children do as we do, not as we say. According to the U.S. Centers for Disease Control and Prevention, nearly three-quarters of U.S. adults eat vegetables fewer than three times per day, the minimum recommended number. And yet vegetables are a key component in the diet of all growing kids, and are crucial for healthy digestion. Veggies are a great source of both soluble and insoluble fiber, and contain a lot less sugar than most fruit (an excellent source of micronutrients and fiber that is also generally more appetizing to young children than the green stuff). However, this doesn't always have to be the case. With a little planning and creativity you can find ways to keep vegetables on the menu and your kids happy and healthy at the same time.

Tips and Tricks for Getting the Whole Family to Eat More Vegetables

Luckily, there are a lot of good, tried-and-true strategies you can use to get everyone in the family back on track when it comes to eating the right foods for digestive health.

◉ **Stay cool.** Even though it may seem a little counterintuitive, staying neutral about the veggies you serve to your kids is a better strategy than bribing or threatening them. Just prepare vegetables in a variety of different ways and serve them without any fanfare. Telling your kids that you're giving them something new, healthy, or otherwise good for them will actually make them less likely to taste it. Just put one new vegetable on the plate with at least one other food you know your child likes and don't say anything about it. Then keep trying. Just be patient and keep putting the vegetable on the plate from time to time, even if your child keeps ignoring or rejecting it. It can take up to fifteen offerings before a young child will actually try something new.

◉ **Capitalize on positive peer pressure.** If kids see their friends eating something, they're much more likely to eat it too. Seeing even one friend eating a salad can help your child give it a try. Serve raw or steamed veggies crudités-style on a playdate, and watch your finicky child follow suit when a friend samples a pretty carrot stick.

- **Hide them!** If your child won't touch a veggie with a ten-foot pole, start by making them "invisible." Puree and mix them into meatballs, meatloaf, or spaghetti sauce. Be sure to match veggie colors with the food you're preparing so that the good stuff stays hidden.

- **Shred and bake.** Grated vegetables can easily be tucked into almost any baked goods. Try hiding zucchini, carrots, and sweet potatoes in muffins, cakes, and even cookies.

- **Finger food, dips, and sprinkles.** Offer veggies "kid-sized," such as individual mini broccoli "trees" or baby carrots. Let your kids dress up plain veggies with their own dips and sauces. A little dipping bowl of creamy homemade salad dressing or a colorful shaker of ground sesame seeds can turn something simple into something special.

- **Be aware of texture.** Some children are very sensitive to the texture of foods, not just to their flavor. It may be that your toddler is refusing a whole category of foods because they don't feel good in the mouth. Try changing the texture of a vegetable your child won't eat to see if that makes a difference. For instance, if your child doesn't like mashed sweet potato or cauliflower, try baked sweet potato "fries" and raw cauliflower florets (with dip, of course!). If your toddler doesn't like to eat anything crunchy just yet, try offering one or two choices of food in the preferred style, while also offering one crispy choice alongside. If the crunchy food can be dipped into something soft and creamy, it just might get eaten. Or vice versa!

- **Bridge with the familiar.** Try offering a new veggie served in exactly the same way as one your child already likes, such as homemade, baked sweet potato "fries" cut like restaurant-style French fries. This familiar presentation will be comforting and may help your child feel a little more secure about trying something new.

- **Keep it simple.** Don't overwhelm your toddler with too many new foods at once. He will generally do better with only two to four offerings on his plate, and only one of those offerings should be something new at any given meal. Kids generally prefer simply prepared foods instead of "mixed-up" foods like casseroles, so try serving very small portions of pretty, recognizable foods in separate areas on the plate. Using a divided plate or three small colored bowls can work magic for some kids who don't want their foods "touching."

◉ **Roast 'em sweet.** Roasting root veggies (carrots, beets, winter squash, etc.) caramelizes the sugars and makes them taste like nature's candy. Try roasting greens, too (such as asparagus, kale, and Brussels sprouts) for an appealing, crispy/chewy texture and a beguiling sweet flavor.

◉ **Make the kitchen a welcoming place.** Encourage your kids to get involved with veggie selection and preparation. For example, ask your kids to help wash salad veggies or arrange them in a pretty way on a platter. If they participate in any phase of meal preparation they are much more likely to actually eat the food they helped to prepare.

◉ **Make your own.** To engage older toddlers, let them customize their meals by setting up a "bar" where they can decorate their own pizzas, salads, or even soup with an assortment of diced or shredded vegetables that they can sprinkle on top. Finely diced greens might actually get sprinkled on a pizza, while a big pile of steamed kale will probably get a howling rejection.

◉ **Make an example.** Clipping photos of kids eating certain foods and hanging them on the fridge or making a chart with them can help picky toddlers visualize eating those foods, so it is more likely that they will actually eat them.

Medicine Cabinet Must-Haves

It is a good idea to have a selection of a few, simple, natural digestive soothers in your medicine cabinet to use when your infant, toddler, or young child has a gastrointestinal complaint. You can easily find safe, effective products in natural-food stores or online. With these products readily on hand, you will be ready for any digestive complaint that may arise.

Probiotics. For constipation, diarrhea, gas and bloating, allergies, and eczema, the dose is ⅛–¼ teaspoon twice daily.

Digestive enzymes. For gas and bloating, food sensitivities, constipation and diarrhea, colic/reflux, and to improve digestive function, give toddlers a pinch of powdered enzymes with meals. For children who can swallow pills, the dose is one capsule with meals.

DGL. This product is often found in wafer form and is wonderful for colic/reflux, indigestion, and a wide range of other digestive complaints. Children can take a chewable wafer after meals. For more information about using DGL to treat colic/reflux, see page 268.

Chamomile Tea. Indigestion, gas, bloating, restlessness and anxiety, colic, and reflux can be relieved with a serving of chamomile tea.

Gripe water. Children can take 10–30 drops of gripe water with meals to reduce the symptoms of colic, reflux, and silent reflux. See page 266 for complete details about these conditions and their treatment.

Slippery elm powder. The dose for stomach pain, diarrhea, constipation, and indigestion is 1–2 teaspoons of slippery elm powder mixed into water, 2–3 times daily.

Encapsulated peppermint oil. Children who can swallow pills should take one capsule after meals for gas/spasm and stomach pain. Note that mint is not appropriate for children who have reflux.

After your child is the age of five or so, you can incorporate bitter herbs, such as milk thistle and dandelion, into a child's diet, in the form of teas, as bitter herbs help support the liver and regulate peristalsis (the rhythmic contraction of the intestines that helps move food down and out through the system). Honey can be added to these strong-flavored teas to improve their taste (although no raw honey should be given to children under the age of two, because honey can contain harmful bacteria). Typically, it is safe to give teas to even very small children, and it is also a great way to increase hydration.

Glossary

Absorption: the act of nutritive particles such as amino acids, fatty acid, sugars, vitamins, minerals, and other compounds traveling from the digestive tract into the blood.

Antibody: an immune particle that is made by the immune cells to bind and neutralize antigens.

Antigen: an antigen is any particle that is not recognized by the body as "self."

Assimilation: the act of absorbed nutritive particles being taken up by cells in order to be incorporated into the body and utilized for metabolism and other bodily functions.

Atopy: the cluster of diseases characterized by environmental allergies, food allergies, eczema, and asthma. These conditions are typically driven by IgE and often occur together.

Autoimmunity: when the immune system makes antibodies and attacks the cells of the body. There are a wide variety of autoimmune conditions, including celiac disease, rheumatoid arthritis, Sjogren's syndrome, Raynaud's disease, lupus, multiple sclerosis, myasthenia gravis, and inflammatory bowel disease.

Autonomic nervous system (ANS): part of the nervous system that acts like the control panel, affecting heart rate, digestion, respiratory rate, salivation, arousal, etc. It is divided into two branches—the sympathetic branch, also known as the "fight or flight" branch, which is dominant in stress situations, and the parasympathetic branch, also known as the "rest and digest" branch, which is important for healthy digestion. Imbalances within the ANS can cause digestive disturbance, sleep issues, and metabolic damage.

Bolus: food that has been chewed and swallowed and ends up in the stomach to be mixed with digestive factors to form chyme.

Casein: the protein molecule that is found in most milk products. Casein is a common food allergen.

Caseomorphin: an intermediate compound created during the digestion of casein-containing foods that binds to opioid receptors in the gut, leaving one wanting more.

Chyme: the semisolid/liquid state of the bolus after it has been mixed with digestive acid, enzymes, and other factors in the stomach.

Desmosome: the button-like anatomical structure that is in between the cells that line the small intestine, helping them stay very close together, and effectively buttoning them together. Certain foods, substances, and stresses can unbutton the desmosome, creating a condition called leaky gut.

Detoxification: the process by which products of metabolism and ingested, inhaled, or absorbed toxic compounds are rendered safer and excreted. This process occurs around the clock. The major organs of detoxification are the liver, kidneys, skin, lungs, and large intestine

Digestion: the multistep process of consuming food, breaking it down, absorbing it into the blood, and assimilating it into the cells and organs of the body

Enteric nervous system (ENS): the so-called second brain, the ENS has as much nervous tissue as the spinal cord. The ENS helps regulate digestive function independent of the brain and central nervous system, although it can communicate with it.

Gluten: the protein found in wheat, barley, rye, and other grains. The gluten molecule in the Unites States has changed over the last couple of decades via aggressive hybridization and is now inflammatory and allergenic.

Gluteomorphin: the intermediate compound created during the digestion of gluten-containing foods that binds to opiod receptors in the gut, leaving one wanting more.

Goitrogen: any substance that can damage the thyroid and lower thyroid function.

IgA: a non-inflammatory immune molecule that coats the lining of the entire digestive tract and genitourinary tract. It acts as one of the first lines of defense against invading pathogens.

IgE: an inflammatory molecule known as the "evil" antibody that is responsible for rapid, acute symptoms of food sensitivity that can potentially be life threatening. IgE food allergy is typically tested via skin-prick testing. People with environmental allergies, asthma, and eczema often have high levels of IgE

IgG: an inflammatory immune molecule that is present when the immune

system has been exposed to foods or other particles that trigger antibody production. High amounts of IgG to foods demonstrate food sensitivity. IgG is responsible for delayed onset, slower acting, not life threatening but chronic symptoms from eating foods one is sensitive to. IgG is detected by blood tests.

Leaky gut: intestinal hyperpermeability, in which the lining of the small instestine is overpermeable and overinflamed.

Molecular mimicry: if the immune system is making antibodies against foods, it is possible for the immune system to then make antibodies against proteins or cells in the body that "look" similar to the foods that the immune system is making antibodies to. This is the mechanism by which food sensitivities and leaky gut can trigger autoimmunity.

Mucosa: also known as the mucous membrane, this is the lining of the entire GI tract.

Peristalsis: the rhythmic, muscular contraction of the intestines that propels food down and through the digestive system, bringing the digested food from the stomach all the way to the toilet.

Tight junction: a closely associated area between two cells, as in the cells that line the small intestine. Tight junctions, along with desmosomes, help keep the integrity of the small intestine intact.

Tolerization: the process by which the immune system is schooled to not attack the cells of the body and the foods consumed. When tolerization is lost, food sensitivities and autoimmune disease may follow.

Sources

Section I:

Ammann R, Kashiwagi H, "Pancreatic exocrine insufficiency and proteolytic enzymes in stool. A critical evaluation of a new diagnostic test in various forms of steatorrhea," *Helv Med Acta.* 33(3) (1966):220-8.

Ayazi S, Tamhankar A, DeMeester SR, Zehetner J, Wu C, Lipham JC, Hagen JA, DeMeester TR, "The impact of gastric distension on the lower esophageal sphincter and its exposure to acid gastric juice," *Ann Surg.* 252(2010):57-62.

Bassotti G, Villanacci V, "Can "functional" constipation be considered as a form of enteric neuro-gliopathy?" *Glia* 59(3) (2011):345-50.

Bellinger DC, "Prenatal Exposures to Environmental Chemicals and Children's Neurodevelopment: An Update," *Saf Health Work.* 4(1) (2013):1-11.

Brelian D, Tenner S, "Diarrhoea due to pancreatic diseases," *Best Pract Res Clin Gastroenterol.* 26(5) (2012):623-31.

Chen J, Zhou X, Zhang Y, Zi Y, Qian Y, Gao H, Lin S, "Binding of triclosan to human serum albumin: insight into the molecular toxicity of emerging contaminant," *Environ Sci Pollut Res Int.* 19(7) (2011):2528-36.

Cirillo C, Vanden Berghe P, Tack J, "Role of serotonin in gastrointestinal physiology and pathology," *Minerva Endocrinol.* 36(4) (2011):311-24.

Cusick MF, Libbey JE, Fujinami RS, "Molecular mimicry as a mechanism of autoimmune disease," *Clin Rev Allergy Immunol.* 42(1) (2012):102-11.

deFoneska A, Kaunitz JD, "Gastroduodenal mucosal defense," *Curr Opin Gastroenterol.* 26(2010):604-10.

De Winter BY, De Man JG, "Interplay between inflammation, immune system and neuronal pathways: effect on gastrointestinal motility," *World J Gastroenterol.* 16(44) (2010):5523-35.

Dodson RE, Nishioka M, Standley LJ, Perovich LJ, Brody JG, Rudel RA, "Endocrine disruptors and asthma-associated chemicals in consumer products," *Environ Health Perspect.* 120(7) (2012):935-43.

Farré R, Tack J, "Food and Symptom Generation in Functional Gastrointestinal Disorders: Physiological Aspects," *Am J Gastroenterol.* 108(5) (2013): 698-706.

Gaby AR, "Nutritional approaches to prevention and treatment of gallstones," *Altern Med Rev.* 14(2009):258-67.

Gao Y, Li X, Yang M, Zhao Q, Liu X, Wang G, Lu X, Wu Q, Wu J, Yang Y, Yang Y, Zhang Y, "Colitis-Accelerated Colorectal Cancer and Metabolic Dysregulation in a Mouse Model," *Carcinogenesis* 34 (2013):1861-9.

Guo LW, Wu Q, Green B, Nolen G, Shi L, Losurdo J, Deng H, Bauer S, Fang JL, Ning B, "Cytotoxicity and inhibitory effects of low-concentration triclosan on adipogenic differentiation of human mesenchymal stem cells," *Toxicol Appl Pharmacol.* 262(2) (2012):117-23.

Kamada N, Seo SU, Chen GY, Núñez G, "Programming of host metabolism by the gut microbiota," *Ann Nutr Metab.* 58 Suppl 2 (2008):44-52.

Kamada N, Seo SU, Chen GY, Núñez G, "Role of the gut microbiota in immunity and inflammatory disease," *Nat Rev Immunol.* 13(2013):321-35.

Konturek SJ, Konturek PC, Pawlik T, Sliwowski Z, Ochmański W, Hahn EG,

"Duodenal mucosal protection by bicarbonate secretion and its mechanisms," *J Physiol Pharmacol.* 55 Suppl 2 (2004):5-17.

Lahner E, Esposito G, Zullo A, Hassan C, Cannaviello C, Paolo MC, Pallotta L, Garbagna N, Grossi E, Annibale B, "High-fibre diet and Lactobacillus paracasei B21060 in symptomatic uncomplicated diverticular disease," *World J Gastroenterol.* 18(2012):5918-24.

Magrone T, Jirillo E, "The interplay between the gut immune system and microbiota in health and disease: nutraceutical intervention for restoring intestinal homeostasis," *Curr Pharm Des.* 19(7) (2013):1329-42.

Neunlist M, Van Landeghem L, Mahé MM, Derkinderen P, des Varannes SB, Rolli-Derkinderen M, "The digestive neuronal-glial-epithelial unit: a new actor in gut health and disease," *Nat Rev Gastroenterol Hepatol.* 10(2) (2013):90-100.

Pannu MW, Toor GS, O'Connor GA, Wilson PC, " Toxicity and bioaccumulation of biosolids-borne triclosan in food crops," *Environ Toxicol Chem.* 31(9) (2012):2130-7.

Popoff MR, Poulain B, "Bacterial toxins and the nervous system: neurotoxins and multipotential toxins interacting with neuronal cells," *Toxins* (Basel). 2(4) (2010):683-737.

Proal AD, Albert PJ, Marshall T, "Autoimmune disease in the era of the metagenome," *Autoimmun Rev.* 8(8) (2009):677-81.

Proal AD, Albert PJ, Marshall TG, "The human microbiome and autoimmunity," *Curr Opin Rheumatol.* 25(2) (2013):234-40.

Raybould HE, Zittel TT, Holzer HH, Lloyd KC, Meyer JH, "Gastroduodenal sensory mechanisms and CCK in inhibition of gastric emptying in response to a meal," *Dig Dis Sci.* 39 (1994) 105-111.

Sachdeva S, Khan Z, Ansari MA, Khalique N, Anees A, "Lifestyle and gallstone disease: scope for primary prevention," *Indian J Community Med.* 36(2011):263-7.

Sasselli V, Pachnis V, Burns AJ, "The enteric ner-vous system," *Dev Biol.* 366(1) (2012):64-73.

Savage JH, Matsui EC, Wood RA, Keet CA, "Urinary levels of triclosan and parabens are associated with aeroallergen and food sensitization," *J Allergy Clin Immunol.*130(2) (2012):453-60.

Schubert ML, "Gastric secretion," *Curr Opin Gastroenterol.* 19(2003):519-25.

Selmi C, Leung PS, Sherr DH, Diaz M, Nyland JF, Monestier M, Rose NR, Gershwin ME, "Mechanisms of environmental influence on human autoimmunity: a National Institute of Environmental Health Sciences expert panel workshop," *J Autoimmun.* 39(4) (2012):272-84.

Su L, Nalle SC, Shen L, Turner ES, Singh G, Breskin LA, Khramtsova EA, Khramtsova G, Tsai PY, Fu YX, Abraham C, Turner JR, "TNFR2 Activates MLCK-Dependent Tight Junction Dysregulation to Cause Apoptosis-Mediated Barrier Loss and Experimental Colitis," *Gastroenterology* 145 (2013): 407-15.

Tarleton S, DiBaise JK, "Low-residue diet in diverticular disease: putting an end to a myth," *Nutr Clin Pract.* 26(2011):137-42.

Turnbaugh PJ, "Microbiology: fat, bile and gut microbes," *Nature* 487(2012):47-8.

Ventrice P, Ventrice D, Russo E, De Sarro G, "Phthalates: European regulation, chemistry, pharmacokinetic and related toxicity," *Environ Toxicol Pharmacol.* 36(1)(2013):88-96.

Vidyashankar S, Sambaiah K, Srinivasan K, "Dietary garlic and onion reduce the incidence of atherogenic diet-induced cholesterol gallstones in experimental mice," *Br J Nutr.* 101(2009):1621-9.

Wick JY, "Diverticular disease: eat your fiber!" *Consult Pharm.* 27(2012):613-8.

Section II and III:

Allen KJ, Koplin JJ, Ponsonby AL, Gurrin LC, Wake M, Vuillermin P, Martin P, Matheson M, Lowe A, Robinson M, Tey D, Osborne NJ, Dang T, Tina Tan HT, Thiele L, Anderson D, Czech H, Sanjeevan J, Zurzolo G, Dwyer T, Tang ML, Hill D, Dharmage SC, "Vitamin D insufficiency is associated with challenge-proven food allergy in infants," *J Allergy Clin Immunol.* 131(2013):1109-1116.

Asadi-Shahmirzadi A, Mozaffari S, Sanei Y, Baeeri M, Hajiaghaee R, Monsef-Esfahani HR, Abdollahi M, "Benefit of Aloe vera and Matricaria recutita mixture in rat irritable bowel syndrome: Combination of antioxidant and spasmolytic effects," *Chin J Integr Med.* (2012)

Asare F, Störsrud S, Simrén M, "Meditation over medication for irritable bowel syndrome? On exercise and alternative treatments for irritable bowel syndrome," *Curr Gastroenterol Rep.* 14 (2012):283-9.

Batista C, Barros L, Carvalho AM, Ferreira IC, "Nutritional and nutraceutical potential of rape (Brassica napus L. var. napus) and 'tronchuda' cabbage (Brassica oleraceae L. var. costata) inflorescences," *Food Chem Toxicol.* 49 (2011):1208-14.

Benmalek Y, Yahia OA, Belkebir A, Fardeau ML, "Anti-microbial and anti-oxidant activities of Illicium verum, Crataegus oxyacantha ssp monogyna and Allium cepa red and white varieties," *Bioengineered.* 4 (2013).

Beutheu S, Ghouzali I, Galas L, Déchelotte P, Coëffier M, "Glutamine and arginine improve permeability and tight junction protein expression in methotrexate-treated Caco-2 cells," *Clin Nutr.* 32 (2013):863-9

Bourne C, Charpiat B, Charhon N, Bertin C, Gouraud A, Mouchoux C, Skalli S, Janoly-

Dumenil A, "Emergent adverse effects of proton pump inhibitors," *Presse Med.* 42 (2013):53-62.

http://www.cdc.gov/healthyyouth/obesity/

http://www.cdc.gov/ibd/

http://www.cdc.gov/obesity/data/adult.html

Chen J, Chen SY, Lian JJ, Zeng XQ, Luo TC, "Pharmacodynamic impacts of proton pump inhibitors on the efficacy of clopidogrel in vivo-a systematic review," *Clin Cardiol.* 36 (2013):184-9.

Ciesielczyk K, Thor PJ, "Neural control disturbances of the gastrointestinal tract and visceral pain in inflammatory bowel diseases," *Postepy Hig Med Dosw.* 67(2013):304-14.

Costabile A, Kolida S, Klinder A, Gietl E, Bäuerlein M, Frohberg C, Landschütze V, Gibson GR, "A double-blind, placebo-controlled, cross-over study to establish the bifidogenic effect of a very-long-chain inulin extracted from globe artichoke (Cynara scolymus) in healthy human subjects," *Br J Nutr.* 104 (2010):1007-17.

Curcic MG, Stankovic MS, Radojevic ID, Stefanovic OD, Comic LR, Topuzovic MD, Djacic DS, Markovic SD, "Biological effects, total phenolic content and flavonoid concentrations of fragrant yellow onion (Allium flavum L.)," *Med Chem.* 8 (2011):46-51.

de Aguiar Vallim TQ, Tarling EJ, Edwards PA, "Pleiotropic Roles of Bile Acids in Metabolism," *Cell Metab.* 17 (2013):657-69

de Jager CP, Wever PC, Gemen EF, van Oijen MG, van Gageldonk-Lafeber AB, Siersema PD, Kusters GC, Laheij RJ, "Proton pump inhibitor therapy predisposes to community-acquired Streptococcus pneumoniae pneumonia," *Aliment Pharmacol Ther.* 36 (2012):941-9.

DebMandal M, Mandal S, "Coconut (Cocos nucifera L.: Arecaceae): in health promotion and disease prevention," *Asian Pac J Trop Med.* 4 (2011):241-7.

Doerge DR, Sheehan DM, "Goitrogenic and estrogenic activity of soy isoflavones," *Environ Health Perspect.* 110 (2002):S349-53.

Escudero C, Sánchez-García S, Rodríguez Del Río P, Pastor-Vargas C, García-Fernández C, Pérez-Rangel I, Ramírez-Jiménez A, Ibáñez MD, "Dehydrated egg white: An allergen source for improving efficacy and safety in the diagnosis and treatment for egg allergy," *Pediatr Allergy Immunol.* 24 (2013):263-9.

Esquenazi D, Wigg MD, Miranda MM, Rodrigues HM, Tostes JB, Rozental S, da Silva AJ, Alviano CS, "Antimicrobial and antiviral activities of polyphenolics from Cocos nucifera Linn. (Palmae) husk fiber extract," *Res Microbiol.* 153 (2002):647-52.

Fahey JW, Wehage SL, Holtzclaw WD, Kensler TW, Egner PA, Shapiro TA, Talalay P, "Protection of humans by plant glucosinolates: efficiency of conversion of glucosinolates to isothiocyanates by the gastrointestinal microflora," *Cancer Prev Res (Phila).* 5 (2012):603-11.

Fasano A, "Leaky gut and autoimmune diseases," *Clin Rev Allergy Immunol.* 42 (2012):71-8.

Fasano A, "Zonulin and its regulation of intestinal barrier function: the biological door to inflammation, autoimmunity, and cancer," *Physiol Rev.* 91 (2011):151-7

Fasano A, "Zonulin, regulation of tight junctions, and autoimmune diseases," *Ann N Y Acad Sci.* 1258 (2012):25-33.

Feinle-Bisset C, Azpiroz F, "Dietary and lifestyle factors in functional dyspepsia," *Nat Rev Gastroenterol Hepatol.* 10 (2013):150-7.

Fletcher PC, Schneider MA, Van Ravenswaay V, Leon Z, "I am doing the best that I can!: Living with inflammatory bowel disease and/or irritable bowel syndrome (part II)," *Clin Nurse Spec.* 22 (2008):278-85.

Geevasinga N, Coleman PL, Webster AC, Roger SD, "Proton pump inhibitors and acute interstitial nephritis," *Clin Gastroenterol Hepatol.* 4 (2006):597-604.

Hasan SA, Wells RD, Davis CM, "Egg hypersensitivity in review," *Allergy Asthma Proc.* 34 (2013):26-32.

Høst A, Halken S, Jacobsen HP, Christensen AE, Herskind AM, Plesner K, "Clinical course of cow's milk protein allergy/intolerance and atopic diseases in childhood," *Pediatr Allergy Immunol.* 13 (2002):S23-8.

Høst A, Jacobsen HP, Halken S, Holmenlund D, "The natural history of cow's milk protein allergy/intolerance," *Eur J Clin Nutr.* 49 (1995):S13-8.

Howell MD, Novack V, Grgurich P, Soulliard D, Novack L, Pencina M, Talmor D, "Iatrogenic gastric acid suppression and the risk of nosocomial Clostridium difficile infection," *Arch Intern Med.*170 (2010):784-90.

Husain Z, Schwartz RA, "Food allergy update: more than a peanut of a problem," *Int J Dermatol.* 52 (2013):286-94.

Iablokov V, Sydora BC, Foshaug R, Meddings J, Driedger D, Churchill T, Fedorak RN, "Naturally occurring glycoalkaloids in potatoes aggravate intestinal inflammation in two mouse models of inflammatory bowel disease," *Dig Dis Sci.* 55 (2010):3078-85.

Inflamm Patel B, Schutte R, Sporns P, Doyle J, Jewel L, Fedorak RN, "Potato glycoalkaloids adversely affect intestinal permeability and aggravate inflammatory bowel disease," *Inflamm Bowel Dis.* 8 (2002):340-6.

http://www.inspirationgreen.com/index. php?q=food-consumption-in-america.html

Iorio RA, Del Duca S, Calamelli E, Pula C, Lodolini M, Scamardella F, Pession A, Ricci G, "Citrus allergy from pollen to clinical symptoms," *PLOS One* 8 (2031):536-80.

Jacobs C, Coss Adame E, Attaluri A, Valestin J, Rao SS, "Dysmotility and proton pump inhibitor use are independent risk factors for small intestinal bacterial and/or fungal overgrowth," *Aliment Pharmacol Ther.* 37 (2013):1103-11

Jacobson MF, "Carcinogenicity and regulation of caramel colorings," *Int J Occup Environ Health.* 18 (2012):254-9.

Kaayla T. Daniel, *The Whole Soy Story* (Washington, DC: New Trends Publishing, 2005)

Karuppiah P, Rajaram S, "Antibacterial effect of Allium sativum cloves and Zingiber officinale rhizomes against multiple-drug resistant clinical pathogens," *Asian Pac J Trop Biomed.* 2 (2012):597-601.

Keefer L, Kiebles JL, Martinovich Z, Cohen E, Van Denburg A, Barrett TA, "Behavioral interventions may prolong remission in patients with inflammatory bowel disease," *Behav Res Ther.* 49 (2011):145-50.

Kjaer HF, Eller E, Andersen KE, Høst A, Bindslev-Jensen C, "The association between early sensitization patterns and subsequent allergic disease. The DARC birth cohort study," *Pediatr Allergy Immunol.* 20 (2009):726-34.

Kobylewski S, Jacobson MF, "Toxicology of food dyes," *Int J Occup Environ Health.* 18 (2012):220-46.

Konishi H, Fujiya M, Kohgo Y, "Traffic control of bacteria-derived molecules: a new system of host-bacterial crosstalk," *Int J Cell Biol.* (2013) doi: 10.1155/2013/757148.

Kuitunen M, Kukkonen K, Juntunen-Backman K, Korpela R, Poussa T, Tuure T, Haahtela T, Savilahti E, "Probiotics prevent IgE-associated allergy until age 5 years in cesarean-delivered children but not in the total cohort," *J Allergy Clin Immunol.* 123 (2009):335-41.

Kwok CS, Loke YK, "Effects of proton pump inhibitors on platelet function in patients receiving clopidogrel: a systematic review," *Drug Saf.* 35 (2012):127-39.

Labus J, Gupta A, Gill HK, Posserud I, Mayer M, Raeen H, Bolus R, Simren M, Naliboff BD, Mayer EA, "Randomised clinical trial: symptoms of the irritable bowel syndrome are improved by a psycho-education group intervention," *Aliment Pharmacol Ther.* 37 (2013):304-15.

Lackner JM, Gudleski GD, Dimuro J, Keefer L, Brenner DM, "Psychosocial predictors of self-reported fatigue in patients with moderate to severe irritable bowel syndrome," *Behav Res Ther.* 51 (2013):323-31.

Langmead L, Dawson C, Hawkins C, Banna N, Loo S, Rampton DS, "Antioxidant effects of herbal therapies used by patients with inflammatory bowel disease: an in vitro study," *Aliment Pharmacol Ther.*16 (2002):197-205.

Leonard CE, Freeman CP, Newcomb CW, Reese PP, Herlim M, Bilker WB, Hennessy S, Strom BL, "Proton pump inhibitors and traditional nonsteroidal anti-inflammatory drugs and the risk of acute interstitial nephritis and acute kidney injury," *Pharmacoepidemiol Drug Saf.* 21 (2012):1155-72.

Leontiadis GI, Miller MA, Howden CW, "How much do PPIs contribute to C. difficile infections?" *Am J Gastroenterol.* 107 (2012):1020-1.

Mahabaleshwarkar RK, Yang Y, Datar MV, Bentley JP, Strum MW, Banahan BF, Null KD, "Risk of adverse cardiovascular outcomes and all-cause mortality associated with concomitant use of clopidogrel and proton pump inhibitors in elderly patients," *Curr Med Res Opin*. 29 (2013):315-23.

Mahmood A, FitzGerald AJ, Marchbank T, Ntatsaki E, Murray D, Ghosh S, Playford RJ, "Zinc carnosine, a health food supplement that stabilises small bowel integrity and stimulates gut repair processes," *Gut* 56 (2007):168-75.

Mallen CD, Mottram S, Wynne-Jones G, Thomas E, "Birth-related exposures and asthma and allergy in adulthood: a population-based cross-sectional study of young adults in North Staffordshire," *J Asthma*. 45 (2008):309-12.

Mandimika T, Baykus H, Vissers Y, Jeurink P, Poortman J, Garza C, Kuiper H, Peijnenburg A, "Differential gene expression in intestinal epithelial cells induced by single and mixtures of potato glycoalkaloids," *J Agric Food Chem*. 55 (2007):10055-66.

Martinez-Medina M, Denizot J, Dreux N, Robin F, Billard E, Bonnet R, Darfeuille-Michaud A, Barnich N, "Western diet induces dysbiosis with increased E coli in CEABAC10 mice, alters host barrier function favouring AIEC colonisation," *Gut* 63 (2014): 116-24.

Marzban G, Mansfeld A, Hemmer W, Stoyanova E, Katinger H, da Câmara Machado ML, "Fruit cross-reactive allergens: a theme of uprising interest for consumers' health," *Biofactors* 23 (2005):235-41.

Matsukura T, Tanaka H, "Applicability of zinc complex of L-carnosine for medical use," *Biochemistry* (Mosc) 65 (2000):817-23.

Morin S, Fischer R, Przybylski-Nicaise L, Bernard H, Corthier G, Rabot S, Wal JM, Hazebrouck S, "Delayed bacterial colonization of the gut alters the host immune response to oral sensitization against cow's milk proteins," *Mol Nutr Food Res*. 56 (2012):1838-47.

Murray MG, Kanuga J, Yee E, Bahna SL, "Milk-induced wheezing in children with asthma," *Allergol Immunopathol (Madr)*. 41 (2012):310-4.

Negele K, Heinrich J, Borte M, von Berg A, Schaaf B, Lehmann I, Wichmann HE, Bolte G, "Mode of delivery and development of atopic disease during the first 2 years of life," *Pediatr Allergy Immunol*.15 (2004):48-54.

Ngamruengphong S, Leontiadis GI, Radhi S, Dentino A, Nugent K, "Proton pump inhibitors and risk of fracture: a systematic review and meta-analysis of observational studies," *Am J Gastroenterol*. 106 (2011):1209-18.

Nilius B, Appendino G, "Spices: The Savory and Beneficial Science of Pungency," *Rev Physiol Biochem Pharmacol*. 164 (2013):1-76.

Nwaru BI, Takkinen HM, Niemelä O, Kaila M, Erkkola M, Ahonen S, Tuomi H, Haapala AM, Kenward MG, Pekkanen J, Lahesmaa R, Kere J, Simell O, Veijola R, Ilonen J, Hyöty H, Knip M, Virtanen SM, "Introduction of complementary foods in infancy and atopic sensitization at the age of 5 years: timing and food diversity in a Finnish birth cohort," *Allergy* 68 (2013):507-16.

Ohama T, Hori M, Momotani E, Iwakura Y, Guo F, Kishi H, Kobayashi S, Ozaki H, "Intestinal inflammation downregulates smooth muscle CPI-17 through induction of TNF-alpha and causes motility disorders," *Am J Physiol Gastrointest Liver Physiol*. 292 (2007):1429-38.

Olivier CE, Lorena SL, Pavan CR, dos Santos RA, dos Santos Lima RP, Pinto DG, da Silva MD, de Lima Zollner R, "Is it just lactose intolerance?" *Allergy Asthma Proc*. 33 (2012):432-6.

Patil H, Lavie CJ, O'Keefe JH, "Cuppa joe: friend or foe? Effects of chronic coffee consumption on cardiovascular and brain health," *Mo Med*. 108 (2011):431-8.

Pearl DS, Masoodi M, Eiden M, Brümmer J, Gullick D, McKeever TM, Whittaker MA, Nitch-Smith H, Brown JF, Shute JK, Mills G, Calder PC, Trebble TM, "Altered colonic mucosal availability of n-3 and n-6 polyunsaturated fatty acids in ulcerative colitis and the relationship to disease activity," *J Crohns Colitis.* 8 (2014):70-9.

Piche T, Ducrotté P, Sabate JM, Coffin B, Zerbib F, Dapoigny M, Hua M, Marine-Barjoan E, Dainese R, Hébuterne X, "Impact of functional bowel symptoms on quality of life and fatigue in quiescent Crohn disease and irritable bowel syndrome," *Neurogastroenterol Motil.* 22 (2010):626-74.

Purohit V, Bode JC, Bode C, Brenner DA, Choudhry MA, Hamilton F, Kang YJ, Keshavarzian A, Rao R, Sartor RB, Swanson C, Turner JR, "Alcohol, intestinal bacterial growth, intestinal permeability to endotoxin, and medical consequences: summary of a symposium," *Alcohol* 42 (2008):349-61.

Raveendra KR, Jayachandra, Srinivasa V, Sushma KR, Allan JJ, Goudar KS, Shivaprasad HN, Venkateshwarlu K, Geetharani P, Sushma G, Agarwal A, "An Extract of Glycyrrhiza glabra (GutGard) Alleviates Symptoms of Functional Dyspepsia: A Randomized, Double-Blind, Placebo-Controlled Study," *Evid Based Complement Alternat Med.* (2012) doi: 10.1155/2012/216970.

Restrepo MI, Mortensen EM, Anzueto A, "Common medications that increase the risk for developing community-acquired pneumonia," *Curr Opin Infect Dis.* 23 (2010):145-51.

Rietjens IM, Martena MJ, Boersma MG, Spiegelenberg W, Alink GM, "Molecular mechanisms of toxicity of important foodborne phytotoxins," *Mol Nutr Food Res.* 49 (2005):131-58.

Salam MT, Margolis HG, McConnell R, McGregor JA, Avol EL, Gilliland FD, "Mode of delivery is associated with asthma and allergy occurrences in children," *Ann Epidemiol.*16 (2006):341-6.

Sarzynski E, Puttarajappa C, Xie Y, Grover M, Laird-Fick H, "Association between proton pump inhibitor use and anemia: a retrospective cohort study," *Dig Dis Sci.* 56 (2011):2349-53.

Targownik LE, Lix LM, Metge CJ, Prior HJ, Leung S, Leslie WD, "Use of proton pump inhibitors and risk of osteoporosis-related fractures," *CMAJ.* 179 (2008):319-26.

Thompson RD, Craig A, Crawford EA, Fairclough D, Gonzalez-Heydrich J, Bousvaros A, Noll RB, DeMaso DR, Szigethy E, "Longitudinal results of cognitive behavioral treatment for youths with inflammatory bowel disease and depressive symptoms," *J Clin Psychol Med Settings.* 19 (2012):329-37.

Tremaroli V, Bäckhed F, "Functional interactions between the gut microbiota and host metabolism," *Nature* 489 (2012):242-9.

Visser J, Rozing J, Sapone A, Lammers K, Fasano A, " Tight junctions, intestinal permeability, and autoimmunity: celiac disease and type 1 diabetes paradigms," *Ann N Y Acad Sci.* 1165 (2009):195-205.

Wood RA, Sicherer SH, Vickery BP, Jones SM, Liu AH, Fleischer DM, Henning AK, Mayer L, Burks AW, Grishin A, Stablein D, Sampson HA, "The natural history of milk allergy in an observational cohort," *J Allergy Clin Immunol.* 131 (2013):805-12.

Yadav M, Jain S, Tomar R, Prasad GB, Yadav H, "Medicinal and biological potential of pumpkin: an updated review," *Nutr Res Rev.* 23 (2010):184-90.

Zhang G, Panigrahy D, Mahakian LM, Yang J, Liu JY, Stephen Lee KS, Wettersten HI, Ulu A, Hu X, Tam S, Hwang SH, Ingham ES, Kieran MW, Weiss RH, Ferrara KW, Hammock BD, "Epoxy metabolites of docosahexaenoic acid (DHA) inhibit angiogenesis, tumor growth, and metastasis," *Proc Natl Acad Sci U S A*. 110(2013):6530-5.

Section IV:

Aditi A, Graham DY, "Vitamin C, gastritis, and gastric disease: a historical review and update," *Dig Dis Sci*. 57 (2012):2504-15.

Alame AM, Bahna H, "Evaluation of constipation," *Clin Colon Rectal Surg*. 25 (2011):5-11.

Ankolekar C, Johnson D, Pinto Mda S, Johnson K, Labbe R, Shetty K, "Inhibitory potential of tea polyphenolics and influence of extraction time against Helicobacter pylori and lack of inhibition of beneficial lactic acid bacteria," *J Med Food*. 14 (2011):1321-9

Asha MK, Debraj D, Prashanth D, Edwin JR, Srikanth HS, Muruganantham N, Dethe SM, Anirban B, Jaya B, Deepak M, Agarwal A, "In vitro anti-Helicobacter pylori activity of a flavonoid rich extract of Glycyrrhiza glabra and its probable mechanisms of action," *J Ethnopharmacol*. 145 (2013):581-6.

Benjamin J, Makharia G, Ahuja V, Anand Rajan KD, Kalaivani M, Gupta SD, Joshi YK, "Glutamine and whey protein improve intestinal permeability and morphology in patients with Crohn's disease: a randomized controlled trial." *Dig Dis Sci*. 57 (2012):1000-12.

Dabos KJ, Sfika E, Vlatta LJ, Giannikopoulos G, "The effect of mastic gum on Helicobacter pylori: a randomized pilot study," *Phytomedicine* 17 (2010):296-9.

Deguchi Y, Andoh A, Inatomi O, Yagi Y, Bamba S, Araki Y, Hata K, Tsujikawa T, Fujiyama Y, "Curcumin prevents the development of dextran sulfate Sodium (DSS)-induced experimental colitis." *Dig Dis Sci*. 52 (2007):2993-8

Dreux N, Denizot J, Martinez-Medina M, Mellmann A, Billig M, Kisiela D, Chattopadhyay S, Sokurenko E, Neut C, Gower-Rousseau C, Colombel JF, Bonnet R, Darfeuille-Michaud A, Barnich N, "Point mutations in FimH adhesin of Crohn's disease-associated adherent-invasive Escherichia coli enhance intestinal inflammatory response," *PLOS Pathog*. (2013) doi: 10.1371/journal.ppat.1003141.

Drummond L, Gearry RB, "Kiwifruit modulation of gastrointestinal motility," *Adv Food Nutr Res*. 68 (2013):219-32.

Dukas L, Willett WC, Giovannucci EL, "Association between physical activity, fiber intake, and other lifestyle variables and constipation in a study of women," *Am J Gastroenterol*. 98 (2003):1790-6.

Epstein J, Docena G, MacDonald TT, Sanderson IR, "Curcumin suppresses p38 mitogen-activated protein kinase activation, reduces IL-1beta and matrix metalloproteinase-3 and enhances IL-10 in the mucosa of children and adults with inflammatory bowel disease." *Br J Nutr*.103 (2010):824-32.

Eswaran S, Muir J, Chey WD, "Fiber and Functional Gastrointestinal Disorders," *Am J Gastroenterol*. 108 (2013):718-27

Green Peter, *Celiac Disease: A Hidden Epidemic* (New York: Harper Collins Publishing, 2010)

Gregori D, Gafare CE, "Multifunctional food: medical evidence and methodological notes on substantiating health claims," *Int J Food Sci Nutr*. 63 (2012):29-36.

Hagen KB, Dagfinrud H, Moe RH, Østerås N, Kjeken I, Grotle M, Smedslund G, "Exercise therapy for bone and muscle health: an overview of systematic reviews," *BMC Med*. 10 (2012):167.

Hale LP, Greer PK, Trinh CT, Gottfried MR, "Treatment with oral bromelain decreases colonic inflammation in the IL-10-deficient murine model of inflammatory bowel disease." *Clin Immunol*. 126 (2008):345-52

Haniadka R, Saldanha E, Sunita V, Palatty PL, Fayad R, Baliga MS, "A review of the gastroprotective effects of ginger (Zingiber officinale Roscoe)," *Food Funct*. 4 (2013):845-55.

Hawrelak JA, Myers SP, "Effects of two natural medicine formulations on irritable bowel syndrome symptoms: a pilot study," *J Altern Complement Med*. 16 (2010):1065-71.

Hering NA, Schulzke JD, "Therapeutic options to modulate barrier defects in inflammatory bowel disease," *Dig Dis*. 27 (2009):450-4

Hollon JR, Cureton PA, Martin ML, Puppa EL, Fasano A, "Trace gluten contamination may play a role in mucosal and clinical recovery in a subgroup of diet-adherent nonresponsive celiac disease patients," *BMC Gastroenterol*. 13 (2013):40.

Hwang JS, Im CR, Im SH, "Immune disorders and its correlation with gut microbiome," *Immune Netw*. 12 (2012):129-38.

Iversen MD, Brawerman M, Iversen CN, "Recommendations and the state of the evidence for physical activity interventions for adults with rheumatoid arthritis: 2007 to present," *Int J Clin Rheumtol*. 7 (2012):489-503.

Jawhara S, Habib K, Maggiotto F, Pignede G, Vandekerckove P, Maes E, Dubuquoy L, Fontaine T, Guerardel Y, Poulain D, "Modulation of intestinal inflammation by yeasts and cell wall extracts: strain dependence and unexpected anti-inflammatory role of glucan fractions," *PLOS One* 7 (2012):e40648.

Jawhara S, Poulain D, "Saccharomyces boulardii decreases inflammation and intestinal colonization by Candida albicans in a mouse model of chemically-induced colitis," *Med Mycol*. 45 (2007):691-700.

Langner E, Greifenberg S, Gruenwald J, "Ginger: history and use," Adv Ther. 15 (1998):25-44.

Liang RY, Wu W, Huang J, Jiang SP, Lin Y, "Magnesium Affects the Cytokine Secretion of CD4(+) T Lymphocytes in Acute Asthma," J Asthma 49 (2012):1012-5.

Lionetti E, Castellaneta S, Pulvirenti A, Tonutti E, Francavilla R, Fasano A, Catassi C, "Prevalence and natural history of potential celiac disease in at-family-risk infants prospectively investigated from birth," *J Pediatr*. 161 (2012):908-14.

Markland AD, Palsson O, Goode PS, Burgio KL, Busby-Whitehead J, Whitehead WE, "Association of Low Dietary Intake of Fiber and Liquids With Constipation: Evidence From the National Health and Nutrition Examination Survey," *Am J Gastroenterol*. 108 (2013):796-803

Meriga B, Mopuri R, MuraliKrishna T, "Insecticidal, antimicrobial and antioxidant activities of bulb extracts of Allium sativum," *Asian Pac J Trop Med*. 5 (2012):391-5.

Murzyn A, Krasowska A, Stefanowicz P, Dziadkowiec D, Łukaszewicz M, "Capric acid secreted by S. boulardii inhibits C. albicans filamentous growth, adhesion and biofilm formation," *PLOS One* 5 (2010):120-50.

Onken JE, Greer PK, Calingaert B, Hale LP, "Bromelain treatment decreases secretion of pro-inflammatory cytokines and chemokines by colon biopsies in vitro." *J Altern Complement Med*. 15 (2009):891-7

Pietzak M, "Celiac disease, wheat allergy, and gluten sensitivity: when gluten free is not a fad," *J Parenter Enteral Nutr*. 36 (2012):68S-75S.

Pirotta M, "Irritable bowel syndrome—The role of complementary medicines in treatment," *Aust Fam Physician*. 38 (2009):966-8.

Pyleris E, Giamarellos-Bourboulis EJ, Tzivras D, Koussoulas V, Barbatzas C, Pimentel M, "The prevalence of overgrowth by aerobic bacteria in the small intestine by small bowel culture: relationship with irritable bowel syndrome," *Dig Dis Sci*. 57 (2012):1321-9.

Rosania R, Giorgio F, Principi M, Amoruso A, Monno R, Di Leo A, Ierardi E, "Effect of probiotic or prebiotic supplementation on antibiotic therapy in the small intestinal bacterial overgrowth: a comparative evaluation," *Curr Clin Pharmacol*. 8 (2013):169-72.

Rossi F, Bellini G, Tolone C, Luongo L, Mancusi S, Papparella A, Sturgeon C, Fasano A, Nobili B, Perrone L, Maione S, del Giudice EM, "The cannabinoid receptor type 2 Q63R variant increases the risk of celiac disease: implication for a novel molecular biomarker and future therapeutic intervention," *Pharmacol Res*. 66 (2011):88-94.

Sainsbury A, Ford AC, "Treatment of irritable bowel syndrome: beyond fiber and antispasmodic agents," *Therap Adv Gastroenterol*. 4 (2011):115-27.

Sapone A, Bai JC, Ciacci C, Dolinsek J, Green PH, Hadjivassiliou M, Kaukinen K, Rostami K, Sanders DS, Schumann M, Ullrich R, Villalta D, Volta U, Catassi C, Fasano A, "Spectrum of gluten-related disorders: consensus on new nomenclature and classification," *BMC Med*. 10 (2012):13.

Secor ER Jr, Shah SJ, Guernsey LA, Schramm CM, Thrall RS, "Bromelain limits airway inflammation in an ovalbumin-induced murine model of established asthma," *Altern Ther Health Med*. 18 (2012):9-17.

Simrén M, Barbara G, Flint HJ, Spiegel BM, Spiller RC, Vanner S, Verdu EF, Whorwell PJ, Zoetendal EG, "Intestinal microbiota in functional bowel disorders: a Rome foundation report," *Gut* 62 (2013):159-76.

Stoicescu A, Andrei M, Becheanu G, Stoicescu M, Nicolaie T, Diculescu M, "Microscopic colitis and small intestinal bacterial overgrowth—diagnosis behind the irritable bowel syndrome?" *Rev Med Chir Soc Med Nat Iasi*. 116 (2012):766-72.

Stremmel W, Ehehalt R, Staffer S, Stoffels S, Mohr A, Karner M, Braun A, "Mucosal protection by phosphatidylcholine." *Dig Dis*. 30 (2012):85-91

Toh ZQ, Anzela A, Tang ML, Licciardi PV, "Probiotic therapy as a novel approach for allergic disease," *Front Pharmacol*. 3 (2012):171.

Valussi M, "Functional foods with digestion-enhancing properties," *Int J Food Sci Nutr*. 63 (2012):82-9.

Vitale G, Barbaro F, Ianiro G, Cesario V, Gasbarrini G, Franceschi F, Gasbarrini A, "Nutritional aspects of Helicobacter pylori infection," *Minerva Gastroenterol Dietol*. 57 (2011):369-77.

Wald A, "Irritable bowel syndrome--diarrhoea," *Best Pract Res Clin Gastroenterol*. 26 (2012):573-80.

Wald A, Rakel D, "Behavioral and complementary approaches for the treatment of irritable bowel syndrome," *Nutr Clin Pract*. 23 (2008):284-92.

Wei D, Ci X, Chu X, Wei M, Hua S, Deng X, "Hesperidin suppresses ovalbumin-induced airway inflammation in a mouse allergic asthma model," *Inflammation* 35 (2011):114-21.

Weinstock LB, Fern SE, Duntley SP, "Restless legs syndrome in patients with irritable bowel syndrome: response to small intestinal bacterial overgrowth therapy," *Dig Dis Sci*. 53 (2008):1252-6.

Weinstock LB, Walters AS, "Restless legs syndrome is associated with irritable bowel syndrome and small intestinal bacterial overgrowth," *Sleep Med.* 12 (2011):610-3.

Wittschier N, Faller G, Hensel A, "Aqueous extracts and polysaccharides from liquorice roots (Glycyrrhiza glabra L.) inhibit adhesion of Helicobacter pylori to human gastric mucosa," *J Ethnopharmacol.* 125 (2009):218-23.

Xu C, Ruan XM, Li HS, Guo BX, Ren XD, Shuang JL, Zhang Z, "Anti-adhesive effect of an acidic polysaccharide from Aloe vera L. var. chinensis (Haw.) Berger on the binding of Helicobacter pylori to the MKN-45 cell line," *J Pharm Pharmacol.* 62 (2010):1753-9.

Yoon SL, Grundmann O, Koepp L, Farrell L, "Management of irritable bowel syndrome (IBS) in adults: conventional and complementary/alternative approaches," *Altern Med Rev.* 16 (2011):134-51.

Section V:

Azad MB, Konya T, Maughan H, Guttman DS, Field CJ, Sears MR, Becker AB, Scott JA, Kozyrskyj AL, "Infant gut microbiota and the hygiene hypothesis of allergic disease: impact of household pets and siblings on microbiota composition and diversity," *Allergy Asthma Clin Immunol.* 9 (2013):15.

Bae SH, Son JS, Lee R, "Effect of fluid intake on the outcome of constipation in children: PEG 4000 versus lactulose," *Pediatr Int.* 5 (2010):594-7.

Czinn SJ, Blanchard S, "Gastroesophageal reflux disease in neonates and infants : when and how to treat," *Paediatr Drugs.* 15 (2013):19-27.

Dehghani SM, Ahmadpour B, Haghighat M, Kashef S, Imanieh MH, Soleimani M, "The Role of Cow's Milk Allergy in Pediatric Chronic Constipation: A Randomized Clinical Trial," *Iran J Pediatr.* 22 (2012):468-74.

del Giudice MM, Leonardi S, Ciprandi G, Galdo F, Gubitosi A, La Rosa M, Salpietro C, Marseglia G, Perrone L, "Probiotics in childhood: allergic illness and respiratory infections," *J Clin Gastroenterol.* 46 (2012):S69-72.

Dinicola C, Kekevian A, Chang C, "Integrative Medicine as Adjunct Therapy in the Treatment of Atopic Dermatitis-the Role of Traditional Chinese Medicine, Dietary Supplements, and Other Modalities," *Clin Rev Allergy Immunol.* 44 (2012):242-53

D'Vaz N, Meldrum SJ, Dunstan JA, Lee-Pullen TF, Metcalfe J, Holt BJ, Serralha M, Tulic MK, Mori TA, Prescott SL, "Fish oil supplementation in early infancy modulates developing infant immune responses," *Clin Exp Allergy.* 42 (2012):1206-16.

El-Hodhod MA, Younis NT, Zaitoun YA, Daoud SD, "Cow's milk allergy related pediatric constipation: appropriate time of milk tolerance," *Pediatr Allergy Immunol.* 21(2010):407-12.

Furuhjelm C, Warstedt K, Fagerås M, Fälth-Magnusson K, Larsson J, Fredriksson M, Duchén K, "Allergic disease in infants up to 2 years of age in relation to plasma omega-3 fatty acids and maternal fish oil supplementation in pregnancy and lactation," *Pediatr Allergy Immunol.* 22 (2011):505-14.

Ghazavi Z, Namnabati M, Faghihinia J, Mirbod M, Ghalriz P, Nekuie A, Fanian N, "Effects of massage therapy of asthmatic children on the anxiety level of mothers," *Iran J Nurs Midwifery Res.* 15 (2010):130-4.

Inan M, Aydiner CY, Tokuc B, Aksu B, Ayvaz S, Ayhan S, Ceylan T, Basaran UN, "Factors associated with childhood constipation," *J Paediatr Child Health.* 43 (2007):700-6.

Irastorza I, Ibañez B, Delgado-Sanzonetti L, Maruri N, Vitoria JC, "Cow's-milk-free diet as a therapeutic option in childhood chronic constipation," *J Pediatr Gastroenterol Nutr.* 51 (2010):171-6.

Jaber R, "Respiratory and allergic diseases: from upper respiratory tract infections to asthma," *Prim Care*. 29 (2002):231-61.

Koch C, Dölle S, Metzger M, Rasche C, Jungclas H, Rühl R, Renz H, Worm M, "Docosahexaenoic acid (DHA) supplementation in atopic eczema: a randomized, double-blind, controlled trial," *Br J Dermatol*. 158 (2008):786-92.

Kranz S, Brauchla M, Slavin JL, Miller KB, "What do we know about dietary fiber intake in children and health? The effects of fiber intake on constipation, obesity, and diabetes in children," *Adv Nutr*. 3 (2012):47-53.

Lee WT, Ip KS, Chan JS, Lui NW, Young BW, "Increased prevalence of constipation in pre-school children is attributable to under-consumption of plant foods: A community-based study," *J Paediatr Child Health*. 44 (2008):170-5.

Loening-Baucke V, "Prevalence, symptoms and outcome of constipation in infants and toddlers," *J Pediatr*. 146 (2005):359-63.

Loening-Baucke V, Miele E, Staiano A, "Fiber (glucomannan) is beneficial in the treatment of childhood constipation," *Pediatrics* 113 (2004):259-64.

Lucassen P, "Colic in infants," *Clin Evid (Online)*. 5 (2010):201.

Manley BJ, Makrides M, Collins CT, McPhee AJ, Gibson RA, Ryan P, Sullivan TR, Davis PG, "High-dose docosahexaenoic acid supplementation of preterm infants: respiratory and allergy outcomes," *Pediatrics* 128 (2011):71-7.

Marrs T, Bruce KD, Logan K, Rivett DW, Perkin MR, Lack G, Flohr C, "Is there an association between microbial exposure and food allergy? A systematic review," *Pediatr Allergy Immunol*. 24 (2013):311-20.

Metsälä J, Lundqvist A, Kaila M, Gissler M, Klaukka T, Virtanen SM, "Maternal and perinatal characteristics and the risk of cow's milk allergy in infants up to 2 years of age: a case-control study nested in the Finnish population," *Am J Epidemiol*. 171 (2010):1310-6.

Mischke M, Plosch T, "More than just a gut instinct—The potential interplay between a baby's nutrition, its gut microbiome and the epigenome," *Am J Physiol Regul Integr Comp Physiol*. 304 (2013):1065-9

Park C, "Mind-body CAM interventions: current status and considerations for integration into clinical health psychology," *J Clin Psychol*. 69 (2013):45-63.

Paulo AZ, Amancio OM, de Morais MB, Tabacow KM, "Low-dietary fiber intake as a risk factor for recurrent abdominal pain in children," Eur J Clin Nutr. 60 (2006):823-7.

Penders J, Thijs C, Vink C, Stelma FF, Snijders B, Kummeling I, van den Brandt PA, Stobberingh EE, "Factors influencing the composition of the intestinal microbiota in early infancy," *Pediatrics* 118 (2006):511-21.

Quitadamo P, Coccorullo P, Giannetti E, Romano C, Chiaro A, Campanozzi A, Poli E, Cucchiara S, Di Nardo G, Staiano A, "A randomized, prospective, comparison study of a mixture of acacia fiber, psyllium fiber, and fructose vs polyethylene glycol 3350 with electrolytes for the treatment of chronic functional constipation in childhood," *J Pediatr*. 161 (2012):710-15.

Rautava S, Kainonen E, Salminen S, Isolauri E, "Maternal probiotic supplementation during pregnancy and breast-feeding reduces the risk of eczema in the infant," *J Allergy Clin Immunol*. 2012 Dec;130(6):1355-60.

Rosenlund H, Magnusson J, Kull I, Håkansson N, Wolk A, Pershagen G, Wickman M, Bergström A, "Antioxidant intake and allergic disease in children," *Clin Exp Allergy*. 42 (2012):1491-500.

Savilahti E, Kukkonen K, Kuitunen M, "Probiotics in the treatment and prevention of allergy in children," *World Allergy Organ J.* 2 (2009):69-76.

Thomas DW, Greer FR, "Probiotics and prebiotics in pediatrics," *Pediatrics* 126 (2010):1217-31.

Tobias N, Mason D, Lutkenhoff M, Stoops M, Ferguson D, "Management principles of organic causes of childhood constipation," *J Pediatr Health Care.* 22 (2008):12-23.

Wickens K, Black P, Stanley TV, Mitchell E, Barthow C, Fitzharris P, Purdie G, Crane J, "A protective effect of Lactobacillus rhamnosus HN001 against eczema in the first 2 years of life persists to age 4 years," *Clin Exp Allergy.* 42 (2012):1071-9.

Resources

Where To Find The Authors
The Naturopathic Health Clinic of North Carolina
Clinical Practice of Jillian Teta, Keoni Teta and Jade Teta
2522 Reynolda Road
Winston-Salem, NC 27106
336-724-4452
www.nhcnc.com
clinic@metaboliceffect.com

The complete supplement line for the gut restoration program is available through NHCNC. We carry only the purest, highest quality supplements that have been through rigorous third party testing. Not all supplements, nor supplement ingredients, are created equal. We can help you choose what is right for you.

Metabolic Effect
Hormonal Fat loss and Lifestyle Company
Founders: Jade and Keoni Teta
2522 Reynolda Road
Winston-Salem, NC 27106
www.metaboliceffect.com

Fix Your Digestion
Blog and Information Page for Dr. Jillian Teta
www.fixyourdigestion.com
Find Dr. Jillian on Facebook: www.facebook.com/fixyourdigestion
and on Twitter, Instagram and Pinterest @ jillianteta

JillFit Physiques
Body and Mind Transformation Coaching for Women
Jill Coleman, Owner
www.jillfit.com

Jeannette Bessinger, The Clean Food Coach™
Additional recipe, menu and clean food cooking resources, including allergen-free, paleo and slow carb specialties
Find Jeannette on Facebook: www.facebook.com/pages/The-Clean-Food-Coach and on Twitter, Instagram and Pinterest @cleanfoodcoach
www.thecleanfoodcoach.com
www.cleanfoodcentral.com

Lifestyle by Poliquin
Fitness and Nutrition Information, Resources, Articles and Recipes
http://www.lifestylebypoliquin.com/

Jonny Bowden—The Rogue Nutritionist
Dishing up diet and lifestyle facts to blow your mind
www.jonnybowden.com

Support Groups
Gluten Intolerance Group
15110 10 Ave SW, Suite A
Seattle, WA 98166
www.gluten.net
info@gluten.net

Celiac Disease Foundation
13251 Ventura Blvd Suite 1
Studio City, CA 91604
www.celiac.org
cdf@celiac.org

Celiac Sprue Association
PO Box 31700
Omaha, NE 68131
www.csaceliacs.org
celiacs@csaceliacs.org

American Celiac Society
PO Box 23455
New Orleans, LA 70183-0455
www.americanceliacsociety.org
americanceliacsociety@yahoo.net

Raising Our Celiac Kids (ROCK)
3527 Fortuna Ranch Road
Encinitas, CA 92024
www.celiackids.com

Canadian Celiac Association
5170 Dixie Road Suite 204
Mississauga, ON L4W 1E3
www.celiac.ca

Inflammatory Bowel Disease Support Group
24 Dixwell Ave #118
New Haven, CT 06511
www.ibdsupport.org

Inflammatory Bowel Disease Support Group—Canada and International
PB Box 94074
Toronto, ON M4N 3R1
Irritable Syndrome Association
24 Dixwell Ave, #118
New Haven, CT 06511
www.ibsgroup.org

Irritable Syndrome Association—Canada and International
PB Box 94074
Toronto, ON M4N 3R1

Find a Food Allergy Support Group
www.foodallergybooks.com/links7.htm

Kids with Food Allergies
5049 Swamp Rd Suite 303 PO Box 554
Fountainville, PA 18923
www.kidswithfoodallergies.org

Medical Information
United States National Library of Medicine
www.nlm.nih.gov

National Digestive Diseases Information Clearinghouse (NDDIC)
http://digestive.niddk.nih.gov/

Gluten Free Drugs
www.glutenfreedrugs.com

Drug Side Effects and Interaction Information
www.drugs.com

Laboratories
Genova Diagnostics (CDSA)
www.gdx.net

The Great Plains Laboratory, Inc (CDSA)
www.greatplainslaboratory.com/home/eng/stool.asp

Life Extension—Laboratory and Blood Testing Services
www.lef.org/Vitamins-Supplements/Blood-Tests/index.htm

Metabolic Solutions, Inc
(Offers a variety of breath tests for SIBO, H. pylori, fructose malabsorption, etc)
www.metsol.com

IMMCO Diagnostics
(Specializes in autoimmune testing)
www.immcodiagnostics.com

Publications
Paleo Magazine—for those following paleo/primal lifestyles, autoimmune support
paleomagonline.com

Gluten-Free Living—for those on gluten free diets
www.glutenfreeliving.com

Living Without—for those living with gluten, dairy and other food allergies
www.livingwithout.com

Allergic Living—for those living with food allergies
allergicliving.com

Books

Digestive Wellness (Liz Lipski)—A comprehensive book for all things related to the gastrointestinal system.

Textbook of Functional Medicine (Institute for Functional Medicine)—This tome is the anthem for functional and integrative medicine. We salute this book and all of the authors contained within it.

The New ME Diet/The Metabolic Effect Diet (Jade and Keoni Teta)—A practical approach to weight loss and body change through tailored nutrition and exercise that will leave you feeling full, satisfied and happy.

Mental Health, Naturally: The Family Guide to Holistic Care for a Healthy Mind and Body (Kathi Kemper, MD)—Practical approaches for complete mind-body health for the whole family. *The Holistic Pediatrician* (Kathi Kemper, MD)—Great resource for common ailments of children and adolescents.

Great Expectations: Best Food for Your Baby and Toddler (Jeannette Bessinger and Tracee Yablon Brenner, RD)—A comprehensive resource on raising your baby and toddler to eat clean from birth.

Eat, Drink and be Gorgeous: A Nutritionist's Guide To Living Well While Living It Up (Esther Blum and James Dignan)—Sometimes, you can have your martinis and drink them too.

Celiac Disease: A Hidden Epidemic (Peter Green, MD)—A wonderful guide to Celiac Disease.

Integrative Gastroenterology (Gerard Mullin)—A review of all complementary, alternative and integrative treatments for gastrointestinal complaints and disorders.

The Second Brain (Michael Gershon, MD)—A very interesting account of the enteric nervous system and the impact it has on the body, including disorders related to the ENS.

Other Resources

Dr. Biesecker's—manufacturer of holistic products for those living with inflammatory bowel disease (IBD)
www.drbieseckers.com

Environmental Working Group (EWG)—Information on research and advocacy in the areas of toxic chemicals, agricultural subsidies, public lands and corporate responsibility. They publish "The Dirty Dozen" and "The Clean Fifteen" lists.
www.ewg.org

Skin Deep Cosmetics Database—subset of EWG, this database grades all cosmetics, personal care products and household products based on toxicity, ability to induce autoimmunity and carcinogenic effects.
www.ewg.org/skindeep/

Green Guide—green living tips, product reviews, environmental health news
www.thegreenguide.com

Weston A. Price Foundation—cornucopia of information on nutrition, healthy living, gardening, etc.
www.westonaprice.org

About the Authors

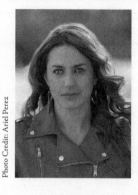

Photo Credit: Ariel Perez

Jillian Sarno Teta, ND, is naturopathic physician and the creator of the Fix Your Digestion gut restoration program, an online, do-it-yourself comprehensive program that can be used by anyone with digestive distress or digestive disorders. Dr. Teta runs coaching groups that enable people with digestive complaints to get to the root of their issues and feel better at www.fixyourdigestion.com.

Dr. Teta received her doctorate in naturopathic medicine from Bastyr University. Before that, she received her Bachelor's and Master's degrees from Boston University in Biology and Energy and Environmental Analysis, respectively.

Dr. Teta practices at the Naturopathic Health Clinic of North Carolina in Winston-Salem and blogs at www.fixyourdigestion.com. She is currently the President of the North Carolina Association of Naturopathic Physicians (NCANP) and a member of the American Association of Naturopathic Physicians (AANP) and Pediatric Association of Naturopathic Physicians (PedANP).

To learn more about Dr. Teta, visit her on Twitter @jillianteta and Facebook www.facebook.com/fixyourdigestion.

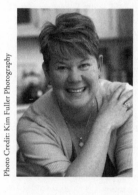

Photo Credit: Kim Fuller Photography

Jeannette Bessinger, CHHC, real food writer, award-winning educator, and chef, is the Clean Food Coach™ (www.thecleanfoodcoach.com). Founder of Clean Food Central (www.cleanfoodcentral.com), an innovative online resource for making faster, tastier meals from seasonal whole foods, she specializes in helping people optimize their eating with less fuss in the kitchen.

Bessinger has designed specialized recipes and meal plans for multiple products, programs, and clean food innovators. She is the author and co-author of eight books that feature healthy eating. Bessinger's work has been showcased in more than 100 media outlets, including *Consumer Reports, Clean Eating, Self, Shape, Better Nutrition, Parenting, Better Homes and Gardens, Redbook, Martha Stewart Living, Dr. Oz Online,* NPR, and NBC News.

The designer and lead facilitator of "Enough Is Enough!", a long-running and successful hospital-based lifestyle-change program, Bessinger acts as a consultant and speaker to national public and private groups and coalitions that are dedicated to improving peoples' diet and health.

Index

Candida, 227–236
   about: overview of, 227
   additional help for, 228–231
   asking doctor about, 231
   causes and symptoms,
      227–228
   constipation and, 193
   dietary interventions, 229
   dysbiosis and, 217–218
   IBS and, 210–211
   lifestyle interventions,
      229–230
   supplements and herbs for,
      230–231
   symptoms of, 66
Capsicum cream, 239–240
Carob in applesauce, 214
Carpeting, asthma and, 234–235
Casein, 43, 74, **288**
Caseomorphins, 43, **288**
Cat's claw, 92
C. difficile infection, 56–57
Celiac disease, 27, 249–254. See
   also Gluten
Chamomile, 92, 184, 269, 271,
   287
Chemical exposure, 45–46
Chewing food, 2, 3, 15–16, 212
Chia seeds, 76
Chicken recipes. See Recipes
   (dinner); Recipes (lunch)
Children. See Kids references
Chlorine, 234, 282
Cholecystokinin (CCK), 13,
   20, 23
Chondroitin, 241
Chromosomes, 39
Chyme, 18, 20, 23, 28, **288**
Cinnamon, 224
Cirrhosis, 23
Citrus fruit, 76, 182, 201
Citrus pectin, 92
Cleaning products, 82–83, 278
Clothing, reflux and, 177
Coconut and coconut products,
   97–98, 139–140, 229, 253, 275,
   279, 280
Coconut sweeteners, 76
Cod liver oil, 204, 275, 280
Colic and reflux in kids,
   266–271
Colitis. See Collagenous
   colitis; Lymphocytic colitis;
   Microscopic colitis; Ulcerative
   colitis (UC)
Collagenous colitis, 198
Colon, characteristics and
   functions, 28
Colonoscopy, 195, 198

Colorectal cancer, 37, 85, 99, 188,
   218, 223
Conditions, about, 175. See also
   specific conditions
Constipation, 185–194
   about: overview of, 185
   additional help for, 188–194
   asking doctor about,
      193–194
   associated conditions, 188
   avoiding/relieving, 212–213,
      274–277, 286, 287
   causes of, 28, 29, 54, 61–64,
      66, 68, 186–188, 273–274
   children and, 271–277
   criteria for, 185
   dietary interventions, 189
   diverticular disease and, 30
   dysbiosis and, 216. See also
      Dysbiosis
   ileocecal valve and, 27
   lifestyle interventions,
      189–190
   not taking time to "go" and,
      29, 187
   nutrition and, 274–277
   ripple effects of, 11–12
   sleep and, 190–191, 273,
      276–277
   supplements and herbs for,
      191–193
   transient, detox and, 103
Corn, 76
Corticosteroids, 54
Cosmetics, 82–83, 278
Cravings, 169–170. See also
   Hunger cues
Crohn's disease, 27, 104, 197,
   198, 201, 202, 205
Cruciferous vegetables, 224
Crypts. See Villi and microvilli
C-section births, 44–45,
   267–268
Curcumin. See Turmeric/
   curcumin

Dairy-free milk, 204
Dairy products, 42–43, 72, 74,
   84, 97, 186, 233, 252, 262, 270,
   272–273
Deglycyrrhizinated licorice
   (DGL), 91, 184, 225, 271, 287
Desmosome, 26, 41, 199–200,
   288
Detoxification, 9–11, 21, **288**.
   See also Liver
Detox symptoms, 103
Dextran sodium sulfate (DSS),
   10, 83, 201

DHA (docosahexaenoic acid),
   38–39, 204, 235, 240, 275
Diabetes, 12, 21, 44, 55, 188, 251
Diarrhea. See also Crohn's
   disease; Irritable bowel
   syndrome (IBS)
   bloody, 196
   causes of, 28, 29, 53, 55, 56,
      65, 66, 68, 179, 209, 223,
      228, 250
   remedies, 202, 212, 262,
      286, 287
   water/electrolyte intake and,
      211
Dietary interventions. See Foods
Dieting. See Metabolic damage/
   weight loss resistance
Digestion
   chewing food and, 2, 3,
      15–16, 212
   defined, **288**
   elimination and. See Bowel
      movements
   organs/players involved in,
      15–32. See also specific
      organs
   process of, 2–4
   transport of food, 3–4
Digestive fire (ability). See also
   Enzymes
   of children, 260, 263
   cholesterol and, 22
   defined, 2
   low, 20, 251
   pancreatic output and, 20
   stoking, 2, 70, 86–89, 181,
      189, 263
Digestive system
   defensive role, 6
   detoxification and, 9–11, 21,
      103, **288**. See also Liver
   impaired, impact of, VII
   roles of, 5–14
Dirt, eating, 45
Diverticulitis, 29, 30, 99
Diverticulosis, 29, 30
Drugs. See Medications and
   digestive health; specific drugs
   and drug categories
Dry brushing, 229
Dysbiosis (bacterial imbalance),
   216–221. See also Bacteria,
   beneficial
   about: overview of, 216
   additional help for, 219–221
   Candida and, 217–218
   causes, types, symptoms,
      216–218
   constipation and, 193